PRAISE

"Drs. Fausz and Howell deliver careful and caring insight into the use of technology, research, and good old common sense to disrupt a stagnant, ailing paradigm and create a healthier healthcare system. Transparent, competitive, and proactive—these ideas mesh perfectly into a world where fitness, both financial and physical, is the goal."

GARY KINDER
United States Olympic Decathlete
Executive Director
Kindersport Human Performance

"Written by two of the most experienced healthcare leaders in the country, this provocative work forces you to consider a new way of looking at our 'sick care' system. And it pushes us to embrace disruption with all its unsettling consequences. Now more than ever, we must rethink the system to improve quality, improve access, and lower the skyrocketing costs. This book will be required reading for my students, and I recommend it to all who are searching for a solution to our broken 'sick care' system."

SUELLYN ELLERBE, MN, RN
Professor, Camden School of Nursing, DNP/MBA Program
Rutgers University

"Although healthcare is both an art and a science, we can clearly learn from corporate models such as Amazon and Walmart how to deliver effective, evidence-based, conscientious healthcare. Authors Fausz and Howell are correct: The time is now. Providers either change or continue to be the conveyor belt in inadequate medical management, and sooner or later each of us and our families will be on that conveyor belt."

EDWARD T. CREAGAN, MD, FAAHPM
Medical Oncologist and Hospice and Palliative Care Specialist
Emeritus Professor of Medical Oncology
Mayo Clinic Medical School

"As W. Edwards Deming said, 'In God we trust, all others must bring data.' Unfortunately, the data show nearly 50 percent of people are suffering from chronic disease despite trillions of dollars spent on healthcare. This is a sad and unsustainable reality that Terry and Aaron powerfully outline while providing a transformative road map for fixing healthcare and encouraging a focus on a vibrant health span instead of a dire life-span."

JOSH JARRETT
Founder and CEO
Quantify Fitness

"Who best to write a book about healthcare transformation than two insiders with years of experience and in-depth knowledge of the inner workings of America's healthcare systems. Terry Howell and Aaron Fausz have outlined innovative solutions to fix America's broken healthcare system that can be applied to both old and new challenges—such as the opioid/substance abuse disorder crisis sweeping America."

RICHARD TAYLOR
Director of Business Development
eTransX Inc.

"Recognizing that healthcare has become trapped in a sick system and a tsunami of disruption is coming, Aaron and Terry offer a way forward. As industry experts, they have experienced firsthand the many obstacles to improving the current system and advocate dramatic changes that will move the system from sick care to healthcare, including systemic innovations that have the potential to truly transform our system of care."

PHILLIP E. GIBBS, PhD
Founder and CEO
The Disruption Lab

HEALTHCARE
IS KILLING
US

The Power of Disruptive Innovation to Create a System that Cares More and Costs Less

AARON FAUSZ, PhD   **W. TERRY HOWELL, EdD**

Skye Solutions
NASHVILLE

Published by:
Skye Solutions Nashville
A division of Skye Solutions, LLC
P.O. Box 366
Thompson Station, TN 37179

www.HealthcareIsKillingUs.com

Hardcover:	978-1-7339325-1-6
Paperback:	978-1-7339325-2-3
Mobi:	978-1-7339325-3-0
EPUB:	978-1-7339325-4-7
Audiobook:	978-1-7339325-5-4

Library of Congress Control Number: 2019938613
Library of Congress Cataloging in Publication Data on file with the Publisher.

Production and design by Concierge Marketing Book Publishing Services

Printed in the United States of America.

10 9 8 7 6 5 4 3 2 1

To those who have suffered too long within the
current sick care system—patients, employers,
and healthcare professionals—as well as to all
who want to imagine and cocreate with us the
reality of vibrant healthcare for all.

CONTENTS

AMERICA'S HEALTH CARE SYSTEM IS NEITHER HEALTHY, CARING, NOR A SYSTEM.

—Walter Cronkite, American broadcast
journalist and nineteen-year anchor
for the CBS Evening News

PREFACE:
Healthcare Is **Killing US**, Physically, Financially, and Spiritually

In 2013 the worldwide fleet of Boeing 787 Dreamliners (a long-haul wide-body jet) was grounded after a number of incidents stemming from its lithium-ion batteries. This lasted 123 days until Boeing completed tests on a revised battery design and the FAA approved it. Not a single 787 had crashed nor was anyone ever injured, but a grounding estimated to have cost over $600 million was undertaken for the sake of passenger and crew safety.

More recently, two crashes of Boeing's 737 MAX—one in 2018 that killed 181 people and one in 2019 that killed 157 people—resulted in the grounding of the world wide fleet of 737 MAX aircraft (the newest version of Boeing's venerable 737 narrow-body jet) until the cause(s) were determined and remedies put into place.

But what if four 737s each carrying 170 people crashed somewhere in the United States and killed everyone on board? Now imagine that happening every day.

Astonishingly, that many preventable deaths happen each day across the various healthcare settings in this country. Yes, the healthcare system is killing us, literally. Every day.

Make no mistake, we're not referring to very sick or those suffering from terminal illnesses who die in hospitals. We're referring to the more than 250,000 people who die each year from preventable medical errors such as the administration of the wrong drug, wrong dose, or a bad combination of medications; from healthcare-associated infections (when medical providers unintentionally infect their patients with something); from blood poisoning; from botched surgeries; and from many other causes.

NOTE: There is no exact count of annual deaths due to medical errors. Studies use various ways to delineate this number, and estimates range anywhere from 200,000 to over 400,000. We've chosen to use the number from research at Johns Hopkins Medicine that took multiple studies and extrapolated from them collectively.

At its current rate (250,000+ per year), healthcare errors are the third leading cause of death in the US after heart disease (635,260) and cancer (598,038). But even more startling is the fact that the problem is most likely being under-reported. Deaths due to medical errors are not currently reported explicitly as a cause of death to the Centers for Disease Control and Prevention, or on death certificates. And they are not easily tracked through the diagnostic and procedural coding system used by hospitals and other providers.

A far more common outcome than death is serious harm, which is estimated to affect 10 to 20 times more patients (6,850 to 13,700 per day) than lethal harm. A study published in *Health Affairs* found that adverse events occurred in as many as one-third of hospital admissions. These errors can result in significant financial, physical, and psychological burdens on patients, who may be left with significant pain or disability.

Deaths caused by drug overdose have been steadily increasing in the US over the past two decades, from an estimated 16,849 in 1999 to just over 70,000 in 2017. That's more Americans than are killed by car crashes (39,000 per year), more than died from AIDS at the height of that epidemic (42,000), and more than were killed during the entire Vietnam War (58,000).

Roughly two-thirds of these needless deaths (approximately 47,600 each year) are due to opioid use. The majority of these began with a patient following doctor's orders taking legally prescribed opioids for pain. Drug companies such as Purdue Pharma aggressively marketed their opioid products as non-habit inducing and moderate (despite there being little to no research to back up these claims), and the healthcare industry responded to these bogus claims by overprescribing these drugs to treat pain. In addition, opioid medications were more widely covered by insurance policies than alternative treatments and therapies, making the drugs an easy choice for everyone.

With an average of 130 Americans dying every day from opioid overdose, let's add a McDonnell Douglas MD-80 crashing and killing everyone on board in the United States every day. How long would we tolerate that?

The unintended, preventable medical errors that occur each year contribute directly to the economic burden of our healthcare system. According to a report by the Commonwealth Fund, the Institute of Medicine (now called the National Academy of Medicine) estimated that medical errors cost $17 billion to $29 billion per year.

In his book *The Opioid Crisis Wake-Up Call*, Dave Chase brilliantly outlines how rising medical costs have largely negated pay raises for the middle class and have even caused an economic depression (defined as two or more years of income decline) among the middle class for nearly twenty years. It turns out that as household incomes were rising by an average of 2.1 percent each year, our health insurance costs were rising by an average of 8 percent each year. Chase goes on to suggest that medical bills may be a leading cause of homelessness, and he reports that nearly half of all GoFundMe crowdfunding campaigns are set up to pay for medical-related expenses.

Chase even presents some very rough, hypothetical calculations for what people could be saving for retirement if it weren't for ballooning healthcare costs. Using historical rates of inflation, performance of the S&P 500 stocks, and healthcare premiums, he determined that over a thirty-year period, the average American household could have saved $1 million in their retirement accounts. Even if his numbers are overstated by 50 percent, $500,000 in retirement savings is a far cry from the next to nothing that the average American household currently has saved.

The percentage of bankruptcies from overwhelming medical expenses garnered splashy headlines for a while, with estimates soaring as high as 60 percent (mainly from politicians citing dubious studies to rally support for their misguided solutions). These numbers were recently debunked by a team of health and labor economists who published the results of a more thorough study in the *New England Journal of Medicine*. They found the number to be only 4 percent.

Correspondingly, we've seen estimates of the number of Americans who declare bankruptcy annually due to medical bills to range from 530,000 to 1.5 million. Even using the lowest of these estimates, medical expenses undoubtedly play a causal role in many personal bankruptcies.

Here are some startling figures from the National Bankruptcy Forum:

» One in ten adults delays medical care due to costs.

» An unexpected $500 medical bill is too much for many people to pay.

» One in five working-age Americans with health insurance has trouble paying off their medical bills.

» More than 60 percent of insured Americans with medical bills spend most or all of their savings on medical expenses.

» Another nearly 60 percent of people who have problems paying their medical bills have been contacted
by a collection agency in the past year.

» While other studies say 4 percent, this forum suggested that some 7 percent of adults struggling with
medical bills have declared bankruptcy.

The healthcare system is also killing us economically at the
state and national levels. Dave Chase presented Massachusetts
as a cautionary tale. In 2006 the state adopted a nearly universal
health insurance program. The increase in healthcare coverage
came with a 37 percent increase in healthcare costs, which
in turn resulted in decreased funding for education (12.2%),
infrastructure (14%), mental health (22.2%), and local aid
(50.5%). In addition, at least some of the hundreds of millions
of dollars in states' unfunded pension commitments can be
attributed to increased healthcare spending.

The healthcare system is choking funding for public education, infrastructure, and social services and, in the process,
stealing the future from our children and grandchildren.

Finally, the healthcare system is killing us spiritually, especially the outstanding medical professionals who toil within
the system every day. *Epidemic, alarming, pervasive*, and *public
health crisis* are just a few of the terms used to describe the
burnout experienced by an increasing number of medical
providers. Although physician burnout receives the most
attention, it is very much an issue for nurses and other medical
providers, so we refer to it here in an all-encompassing sense.

We suspect much of this burnout is caused by the collision of
idealistic hopes and dreams with the administrative and procedural duties imposed by our healthcare system. The mounting
number of administrative requirements have disconnected
medical providers from the reasons they chose healthcare as a
profession in the first place. Nearly every provider we've interacted

with over the years has complained about spending more time performing mundane nonmedical tasks (usually while staring into a computer) than they do interacting with patients. Combined with the uncertainty prevalent in today's healthcare industry and the higher acuity of patients, the environment in which they must practice medicine has become overwhelming.

It's no wonder medical providers feel increasingly burned out. As the manifestations of burnout (exhaustion, depersonalization, diminished sense of accomplishment, etc.) wear down providers' physical, intellectual, and social health, feelings about their chosen profession naturally wane.

Surveys have shown that a large majority of providers are not satisfied with their work and would not even recommend healthcare as a profession. Providers' emotional and psychological health may even become jeopardized, sometimes to the point where providers experience trouble in relationships or become clinically depressed and, in extreme instances, consider suicide.

Burnout at these levels is not good for anyone, especially medical providers entrusted with the care, safety, and health of others.

From our perspective, it is clear that healthcare is killing us in many ways. We agree with Dave Chase, who said "the health care system has become the greatest immediate threat to our freedom to pursue health and the American Dream."

We'll add that a broken healthcare system is the greatest immediate threat to our country's long-term solvency.

IMAGINE

The healthcare industry is killing us physically, financially, and spiritually. But it doesn't have to be this way. Consumers and patients deserve better, and the industry can heal itself to exceed our expectations. We ask that you imagine a different mindset for health and healthcare in the United States:

» Imagine that health and well-being are lifelong pursuits for individuals.

» Imagine a true healthcare system that delivers solutions to improve health—not just treat/manage disease.

» Imagine a healthcare system that addresses patients' physical, social, and emotional circumstances as well as basic resource needs (such as food and shelter) as a routine part of care.

» Imagine that evidence-based information about which diagnostics and therapies work best and how much they cost is readily available to individuals and medical care providers whenever it is needed.

» Imagine that this evidence-based information includes both traditional and alternative methods.

» Imagine a healthcare system that does not center on doctors, hospitals, and drug/device manufacturers, but rather on consumers and their families who are fully capable of making decisions about their health needs because they have been provided with the necessary tools, information, and opportunities.

That's what we think health and healthcare could look and feel like.

So wouldn't it be nice if…

Everyone views staying healthy and living a healthy lifestyle as one of the most important things they can do for themselves and their loved ones. Internalizing the value of health and wellness, parents model healthy behaviors for their children and instill in them a sense of the importance of staying healthy.

Schools reinforce the message of health and well-being, and every student participates in daily physical education. Knowing how fitness positively impacts their lives, professional athletes and celebrities routinely visit schools and youth clubs to spread the word about health and fitness, demonstrate fun exercises, and help convince impressionable youth that being healthy (and staying out of trouble) is cool.

Imagine that everyone walks more and spends more time engaged in physical activity than they do staring at a screen of any sort. Consider the health benefits if stand-up desks are ubiquitous at workplaces and schools, and elevators are only used to go more than five floors.

What if memberships at gyms and fitness clubs are at an all-time high, are busy most of the time, and salaries for fitness/health/strength coaches are comparable to those of other college-educated professions?

Imagine that careers in healthcare—besides doctors and nurses—are more widely known, appreciated, and viewed as excellent occupational choices with above-average compensation.

What if any time a need arises, consumers can easily access the information necessary to make informed choices about health and medical care for themselves as well as for family members/loved ones? What if these decisions are based on meaningful comparative data, not on a physician's or hospital's general reputation, the experiences of friends, or where a physician has admitting privileges? What if consumers know exactly what each physician and hospital across the country charges for standard procedures and what their bill will be so they can make an informed choice?

Imagine that consumers also know the quality scores and safety outcomes for each physician and hospital across the country. In other words, the value proposition of cost/quality/appropriateness is published and kept up-to-date for consumers. With this information, consumers are empowered, able, and financially incented to seek out the most cost-effective care with the best outcomes without worrying about being in or out of network—they can just choose the most affordable care with the best outcomes. In this ideal world, medical providers truly compete for consumers' business.

Imagine that health insurance was rational, made sense, and was affordable for individuals and families. The primary purpose of health insurance is widely acknowledged as covering catastrophic care. Health savings accounts (HSAs) are available to everyone so they can save for the day-to-day, routine expenses individuals are responsible for. Health insurance and HSA contributions are not tied to employment, but widely available at affordable prices in a free (non-government-run) market (like every other form of insurance). Healthy behaviors, healthy lifestyles, and healthy living are encouraged, reinforced, and rewarded with significantly lower premiums.

Imagine that billing for health-related care was straightforward, and bills were clear and easily understood. Consumers do not receive unexpected bills, or bills for services that should have been covered by insurance. Customers pay for routine care like any other commodity—by the consumer making a payment directly to a provider of their choice for an amount agreed upon by both parties in advance (like every other product and service we purchase).

For catastrophic care, health plan copays, deductibles, out-of-pocket maximums, and exclusions are well defined and known in advance. Before making a health-related decision, consumers know exactly what everything will cost as well as which costs they will be responsible for and which costs will be covered by insurance.

Imagine that the cost for prescription medications is transparent, reasonable, and known in advance. Pricing practices on the part of pharmaceutical companies do not harm consumers. Citizens in the United States pay no more than the lowest possible price compared to anywhere in the world, and no longer subsidize the cost of medications for everyone else. Medications are sent to consumers arranged in small envelopes that have exactly what is needed each day so consumers will know if they took the right amount at the right time each day. Instructions for medications are written so people don't need a PhD in chemistry to understand them.

In terms of data and privacy, consumers have complete control over their digital lives, especially as it pertains to their health and health records. No longer are consumers presented with lengthy terms and conditions that give them little choice other than to give up control over their digital footprints. No longer are the technologies and platforms that contain consumers' data—and wield increasing influence over their everyday lives—opaque and largely unaccountable. No longer are health data locked away and exploited by companies for commercial gains. New standards of privacy and control are in place that ensure personal data sovereignty.

Consumers own their data and are empowered by it, and the digital platforms we use help us unlock personal and public benefits with our data by raising awareness and enabling us to take action. With respect to medical records, they belong to consumers—not to providers, hospitals, or insurers—and they go with consumers wherever they are. No longer will consumers have to fill out the same form twice or provide the same information more than once unless their health circumstances change. And a consumer's medical record can be easily accessed and edited by whichever provider they choose.

It is simple and stress-free for consumers to access care when and where it is most convenient for them, including through digital channels like email, apps, social media, and other eHealth platforms using video conferencing/telemedicine. No longer will consumers wait a week for an appointment, experience long waits to see a provider, or nervously wonder which of the people sitting around them in the waiting room are the most contagious.

Imagine a world in which consumers receive routine physicals and checkups using technology in their homes with equipment that monitors vital signs in real time and provides alerts to them and their designated provider if anything needs attention. If face-to-face consultation is required, provider visits to consumers' homes will supplant visits to the office, clinic, or emergency room as the default option. If an office or clinic visit is necessary, a wide selection of choices is available nearby via neighborhood clinics in nontraditional locations (such as retailers, grocers, and workplaces) as well as at provider offices with no appointment necessary and little, if any, wait.

Medical providers think of themselves as—and act like— consumers' health coaches, counselors, and advocates. Providers acknowledge that people's bodies belong to them, not the providers. Providers partner with and include patients (and their families when appropriate) to ensure that that healthiness and well-being are part of everyone's daily routines, to prevent illness, and to jointly discuss and resolve any health issues that arise.

Providers use the most current, scientifically sound information and technology to help diagnose and treat their patients, using an evidence-based approach rather than eminence-based. Providers know as much about nutrition and other healthy interventions as they do about prescribing medications. Since no one can learn everything they need to know in medical school, providers have trouble-free access to artificial intelligence and digital assistants to augment their knowledge and to help with diagnosis and treatment.

Imagine that providers are aware of and consider consumers' socioeconomic situations and basic resource needs when making prevention and treatment recommendations. Providers feel energy and excitement every day as they spend more time with patients and less time performing administrative tasks. Providers have also abandoned white coats so they do not make people feel inferior or delude themselves that they are somehow superior.

If nonemergent inpatient care in a hospital is necessary, patients are greeted warmly and escorted to a room upon arrival. The hospital itself is a place of healing beauty instead of sterile, ugly hallways and rooms. A host orients patients to their room and initiates a reasonable intake/registration process that is typically completed within the first fifteen minutes after arriving in the room.

During the next forty-five minutes a physician-nurse-pharmacist triad performs an initial assessment and confers with the patient to determine a suitable plan of care for the hospital stay. The triad counsels the patient, clearly explains what will most likely happen each day, orders any necessary services, and identifies an estimated discharge date. Any staff member who subsequently enters the patient's room identifies himself or herself, explains what they will be doing and why it is needed, performs their tasks, and asks if the patient has any questions or needs anything else.

Patients are able to order nourishing and healthy snacks/meals a la carte whenever they are hungry. The physician-nurse-pharmacist triad confers with patients daily to view progress, adjust the treatment regimen as necessary, and discuss the discharge process as well as post-discharge instructions with the patient. Before patients leave the room, someone from the care team thanks them for entrusting their care to the hospital and its staff.

If transportation to the hospital or back home or to rehab after discharge is an issue, a ride service is provided as part of the overall cost. The aforementioned items would occur consistently, regardless of the time or day a patient arrives to receive care.

Medical errors have been reduced to zero, and similar to aircraft crashes, any that occur are studied and the findings widely published so that the same error is never made twice. Everyone in healthcare is trained in improvement and innovation, and their mindset is consumer-focused improvement, rapid cycle testing of new ideas, and abandonment of any practice that is not evidence-based and achieving results. A culture of asking questions and continuous learning pervades healthcare organizations. The entire healthcare industry has become a source of rapid cycle testing of new ideas and a place where innovation smoothly follows more innovation.

With proper nutrition and increased physical activity, people are healthier and happier. Life expectancies have increased for all socioeconomic and demographic categories. Gym memberships, fitness boot camps, and healthy restaurants are among the hottest and most profitable businesses. Fast food restaurants have barely survived by introducing more healthy offerings. Junk food sales are sinking steadily, and thanks to pressure by health advocacy groups, the food industry has stopped filling everything with sugar, refined carbohydrates, and antibiotics. The food industry has also stopped lying to the public about which foods are healthy and which are not.

Can you imagine a world in which obesity is declining as people take responsibility for their own health and well-being? Deaths from chronic diseases—including heart disease, asthma, diabetes, and others—are dramatically decreasing and no longer kill or disable more Americans than anything else. Medical providers are financially rewarded for keeping people healthy and out of the hospital, and most have robust, proactive population health programs in place.

Care for the elderly and others nearing the end of their lives is affordable, effective, and humane. Perceptions of aging and end-of-life care have been reframed. The excesses of treatment so pervasive in prior medical practice no longer exist. Palliative care is universally understood and widely used to make end-of-life treatment more compassionate and personal. The care for our country's oldest and sickest patients is loving and dignified. In addition to love, these patients receive companionship and help, making sure they're compliant with provider instructions and advocacy.

Imagine that!

INTRODUCTION

No one could credibly argue that healthcare in the United States is functioning well and not in desperate need of a top to bottom overhaul. Our previous section depicts a perfect world of health and healthcare, but are those goals too lofty? Out of reach? We think not.

We started by pointing out that healthcare is killing us, literally and metaphorically. But this begs a number of questions:

» Why do we allow a system to exist that results in such dire physical, financial, and emotional consequences for us as consumers and patients?

» Why do we allow a system to exist that results in such dire personal and professional consequences for the kind and caring people who work in healthcare?

» Why do we allow a system to exist that results in such dire financial and social consequences for us as a nation?

» Why is the healthcare system so far off the rails? How did it get there? What can and should be done to get it back on track?

Here we will provide some background information about the problems within the healthcare system. We will then preview a sampling of disruptive innovators who have taken note of healthcare's woes and who are beginning to make changes.

We will end with an overview of types of innovation that can (and will) be used to transform healthcare.

As a note to readers, throughout this book we use the terms *medical provider, provider,* and *medical care provider.* All are intended to encompass anyone or any organization that is delivering care to people, including physicians, advance practice providers, nurses, therapists, counselors, technicians, and pharmacists, as well as hospitals, surgery centers, long-term care facilities, and more. Our focus is disrupting the healthcare system as a whole, not to single out one group of professionals or any one type of organization.

WE HAVE SICK CARE, NOT HEALTHCARE

The US does not have a healthcare system. We have a sick care system where medical providers and hospitals are largely paid to treat health problems after they manifest (once people get sick) rather than help people stay healthy. There is less emphasis placed on—and significantly less money earned—helping people stay healthy.

In addition, today's healthcare system treats symptoms, not people. It too often doesn't consider the nonclinical aspects of people's lives that directly impact their health—the physical, social (family and friends, support network, unemployment), financial, and emotional circumstances as well as basic resource needs (such as food insecurity and shelter).

HEALTHCARE IS ANYTHING BUT A FREE MARKET

Our dysfunctional healthcare system does not operate like anything resembling a free market, where consumers are in control and can easily shop around for the healthcare providers who deliver the best service and outcomes at the most reasonable prices. In fact, pricing for most healthcare services and pro-cedures is largely hidden from consumers, not rational, and unexpected bills are common.

The American healthcare system is upside down. The health-care system is not set up for patients nor does it function in their best interests. It is not centered around consumers and patients, but on hospitals, physicians, insurance companies, and the broader medical industrial complex.

THE HEALTHCARE SYSTEM IS SICK

The modern healthcare system has become far too com-plicated, fragmented, wasteful, and frustrating. There is too much inefficiency in the delivery of care. Patients must deal with too many hurdles throughout the course of their care, from making appointments to navigating multiple providers to learning test results.

Further, in spite of all the efforts to move to evidence-based care, too many treatments are eminence-based (that is, suggested by expert physicians who are not to be questioned) rather than evidence-based. This contributes to wide variation in care and a large number of avoidable mistakes, too many of which are fatal. Patients undergo too many unnecessary tests and treatments and are prescribed far too many medications. All of these factors increase waste, increase cost, and decrease quality.

Healthcare has become technocratic, and the human element is frequently missing. It is too often something that is done *to* people rather than in partnership *with* them. Medical providers have been turned into paper pushers and mouse clickers, not the health advocates who were drawn into medicine in the first place, and certainly not the health partners they strive to be (and that patients want).

Few people who touch our existing system—along with many of those working within it—come away feeling good about their experience, much less engaged in the system that supposedly exists to help people. Healthcare has become something that everyone dreads.

TRADITIONAL APPROACHES JUST DON'T WORK

We have been engrossed in attempts to improve the healthcare system for many years, as leaders working within the system and as consultants. Like many of you, we've concluded that the traditional approaches to repairing our ailing system are not working.

The alphabet soup of improvement tools and methodologies (such as TQM, CQI, Six Sigma, and Lean) we've learned, used, and taught over the past three decades have provided only incremental improvement to clinical quality, patient and staff safety, and operational efficiency. And for a number of reasons, healthcare organizations have not been good at sustaining the improvements they have made, as evidenced by the high amount of harm the profession inadvertently inflicts on its customers year after year.

Likewise, cost-reduction initiatives have not provided enduring savings for providers and hospitals, and more tellingly have not reduced costs for consumers. As we described earlier, rising healthcare costs are a major reason for the decline of middle-class wages, when adjusted for inflation, over the last twenty years. Sadly, not only have these efforts been inadequate, they've hardly slowed the rate of cost increases as our population has become sicker. Similarly, more well-intended government programs have not helped; more (and more expensive) drugs have not helped; more (and more expensive) medical equipment has not helped; nor have more (and more complicated and expensive) IT solutions.

HEALTHCARE NEEDS A COMPLETE OVERHAUL

The current healthcare system is fundamentally broken and is in need of a top-to-bottom refurbishment. We're increasingly of the view that it can only be fixed through disruptive innovation. In fact, we believe the healthcare system needs the same level of disruption that companies like VRBO and Airbnb have brought to lodging, Uber and Lyft have brought to transportation, and Amazon and Alibaba have brought to retail. We believe healthcare needs its own Moore's Law, where care advances and costs decline at exponential rates. Nothing else can empower consumers and patients or bring true free-market principles to bear on an industry in so desperate need of transformation.

We've been interested in disruptive innovation for some time and have seen many opportunities for the existing healthcare system to be turned on its head for the benefit of consumers and patients. Given the fervent response we've received from presentations on the topic of healthcare disruption, and with the encouragement of trusted colleagues and friends, we decided the time was right for a book focused on consumer- and patient-centric disruption.

In writing this book, we are singularly interested in helping the healthcare industry create what is best for

» Consumers (to keep them healthy),

» Patients (to help them recover from whatever ails them), and

» The incredible workforce who ceaselessly toil to care for patients who have entrusted their lives to them (to keep staff engaged in meaningful and fulfilling work).

CONSUMERS ARE FED UP WITH HEALTHCARE

Throughout the process of researching and writing this book, we talked to numerous people inside and outside of healthcare about their experiences in receiving care. The response was overwhelming. Everyone had a story (or five!), and most of them were not positive. Healthcare simply has to change, and we believe it will. It will either be changed by those inside the system or, if they don't, and soon, it will be disrupted by those outside the system who not only know how to upend other industries but how to run them better once they take over.

Many naysayers believe the healthcare industry will remain isolated from, if not completely immune to, major changes from outside—regardless of the size, funding, or previous track record of disruption by the challenger. Indeed, healthcare is unlike any other part of the economy. This $3+ trillion industry—approximately one-sixth of the US economy—is governed by a hopelessly snarled mix of payers, administrators, providers, pharmaceutical companies, and manufacturers overlaid by a seemingly limitless web of government regulations.

Think of the opportunity costs. With the money our country has wasted on healthcare, we could have improved our educational system immensely, built badly needed infrastructure, funded scientific exploration, and helped millions out of poverty—not to mention putting money back into the pockets of customers and taxpayers.

To complicate matters even further, the perverse funding of care for most people through employer-based insurance has created generations of people who are unprepared and unable to be diligent consumers of healthcare services and who do not view healthcare as a commodity.

The complexity and fragmentation of the industry—especially the scrambled interactions among insurers, health providers, and

consumers—its opacity, its scale, and the thousands of organizations entrenched in the medical industrial complex who have
a vested (and very lucrative) interest in maintaining the status
quo all combine to perpetuate this dysfunctional system. In
addition, many policies—set by the federal government, state
medical boards, and professional associations—seem expressly
designed to limit consumer options and preserve high costs.

Our experience is that consumers—including us and, we
suspect, most of you—are fed up with the current system. We
are disappointed with many aspects of our healthcare system:
rising and largely unknown costs, difficult access to providers,
increased waiting times, unhelpful consumer-facing technology,
a plethora of time-wasting redundancies, as well as delays in
receiving medical care. Even simple things such as updating a
prescription or requesting a routine appointment have become
overly complicated, time-consuming, and inconvenient.

At the same time, consumers have become accustomed to
doing an increasing array of tasks online. We can easily and
instantly stay current with news and events, communicate with
each other, shop, bank, order groceries and restaurant food to
be delivered, pay bills, and book reservations for travel or meals.
Today's technology-based conveniences are an incredible phenomenon for old and young alike and are quickly being taken
for granted by many. As consumers, we increasingly expect fast,
sophisticated services and products that cater to our needs.

We believe the future of healthcare will be less about the
place where it happens and more about convenience, choice,
cost, and customer service.

THE BARBARIANS ARE AT THE GATE

A number of disruptive innovators see the growing discontent
among consumers and employers regarding healthcare. They see
a system rife with administrative inefficiencies, wide variability

in care delivery, opaque pricing, and customer dissatisfaction. They also see the industry's overall aversion to change. In all of this they see opportunity. Fueled by direct experience with the industry's shortcomings, they are actively questioning the existing paradigm and attempting to fundamentally change the system.

How can we be sure the healthcare industry is ripe for change? Researchers at the University of Pennsylvania's Wharton School of Business examined "common patterns among more recent business model innovations and determined three major signals that an industry could be on the precipice of significant change." These signals were highly regulated, opaque pricing, and dissatisfied customers.

The illustration shows these three signals. It's hard to disagree with their findings that healthcare (along with airlines and real estate) are prime for significant change. In fact, all three industries land in the middle area where these signals overlap.

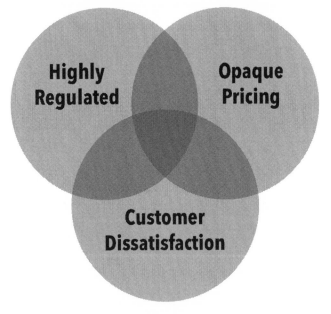

*Three major signals that an industry is
ripe for significant change.*

It's too early to know where any of this will go, how much disruption will take place, who will cause disruption, or how fast it will happen. Google and Microsoft have talked about breaking into healthcare for years, with little to show for it. As of this writing, a few of the proposed ventures are little more than great ideas. However, *something is happening.*

The most successful, forward-thinking, and innovative companies in our country have decided healthcare should be their focus. Given these organizations' track records, their ambitions, and the gaping need for seismic change in the healthcare system, we doubt any of them will create something to fit into the conventional insurance system or more effectively haggle with medical providers over prices. Our bet is they attempt to fundamentally change how healthcare is structured, paid for, and provided. They are trying to disrupt the industry, to make traditional health plans obsolete, and to create a bold new future for American healthcare.

Right now, the biggest mistake any healthcare organization can make is to do nothing. For an industry in such desperate need of change, the biggest risk is standing still.

DISRUPTIVE HEALTHCARE VENTURES ARE MOVING FORWARD

Here is a summary of four of the potentially most disruptive healthcare ventures that have been recently announced. There are others, but these are the most publicized and will give you a flavor for what is coming.

Amazon–JPMorgan Chase– Berkshire Hathaway

This collaboration to build a nonprofit technology-focused healthcare company (subsequently named Haven) was announced in January 2018. Since then, this partnership has mostly kept quiet about its foray into healthcare, but wants to bring down healthcare costs for their US employees and their families. They intend to do this by taking a fresh approach to technology solutions that will help provide simplified, high-quality, and transparent healthcare at a reasonable cost. They will also operate onsite medical clinics for their staff. They will do this on their own, bypassing third-party healthcare organizations.

Their underlying premise is to go beyond just squeezing middlemen by actually lowering costs and delivering better care. It seems likely that the group's initial focus on their own employees' healthcare could be a first step toward impacting the broader US population, a feat that seems reasonable for this large, wealthy, and tech-savvy trio.

While scant information has been shared to date, several key hires were made during 2018. Most significantly, Atul Gawande, MD (surgeon, author, and public health researcher) was named CEO of the new entity. Shortly thereafter, Maulik Majmudar, MD (a cardiologist who was then the associate director of the Healthcare Transformation Lab at Massachusetts General Hospital) was brought on board in an unspecified role. The prevailing assumption is that these two will lead a team of bright people to figure out the details.

Although this partnership has been the most opaque, Amazon founder Jeff Bezos has relentlessly entered new and disparate markets with great success. Amazon has already altered healthcare infrastructure dramatically with Amazon's widely used cloud services and has been trying to expand its healthcare footprint even more. It bought online pharmacy PillPack in early 2018 and is stepping up efforts to sell medical products/supplies to hospitals. Amazon has looked at medical diagnostics, specifically at-home testing, and it filed a patent for its Alexa voice assistant to pick up on a cold or a cough.

Amazon has also started to sell software that will mine patient medical records for information doctors and hospitals could use to improve care and cut costs. In addition, they have many of the core competencies needed to compete in healthcare, including a substantial distribution infrastructure, strong technology base, robust analytics capability, a highly talented workforce, and an incredibly capable leadership team.

Apple

The creator of the iMac, iPhone, and iTunes has already made the use of iOS devices widespread in healthcare organizations. Apple continues to announce different avenues they are pursuing to revolutionize healthcare.

On the consumer side, Apple is actively turning its consumer products into patient health hubs. They intend to move beyond wellness apps and devices by bringing medical records to the iPhone. Over a hundred hospitals have signed on to beta test the new system (with more signing on every week), which aggregates existing patient-generated data with data from the user's EHR (electronic health record).

Patients at participating hospitals will be able to see their own patient history as well as information currently only available in EHR patient portals, such as lab results, hospital data updates, and more. In addition, Apple is undertaking a heart rhythm research project with Stanford University School of Medicine and telehealth vendor American Well.

Apple is also focusing on the health of its own employees with plans to open two company owned and operated clinics in California that will deliver a world-class healthcare experience. Like Amazon, Apple plans to do this without involvement of third-party medical providers. The clinics will have a holistic orientation, staffed by physicians and lab technicians as well as exercise specialists and care navigators. Population health and preventive care will be the guiding principles, intended first and foremost to drive down costs by helping employees and their families stay healthy.

Alphabet/Google
(mainly through a subsidiary called Verily)

Alphabet is focused on leveraging its dominance in data storage and analytics to become the leader in population health. Several recent forays into healthcare signal Alphabet's long-term commitment to industry transformation.

Alphabet is parlaying its broad artificial intelligence (AI) capabilities to address various diseases with an approach centered on using AI for disease detection and disease/lifestyle management. For example, it is working on detecting diabetic retinopathy and combating heart disease, Parkinson's disease, and multiple sclerosis. Alphabet is even planning to tackle COPD, cancer, and behavioral health diseases. Alphabet is also considering the use of AI through products such as Google Home to explore patient-facing health assessments.

In addition, Alphabet has partnered with Johnson & Johnson to build a surgery platform tying together robotics, data analytics, visualization, and more. It is moving into the realm of interoperability solutions with its acquisition of Apigee to help build interfaces that enable one software program to access the services of another. In addition, Alphabet is pushing its Google cloud platform and G suite for healthcare businesses and is developing its own datasets for use in various external research projects.

In a move most related to the current healthcare system, Verily is looking for opportunities to break into the managed care space. It reportedly weighed entering a partnership with a private health insurer on a Medicaid managed care plan in Rhode Island, betting they could administer health insurance more efficiently.

Interestingly, none of these organizations appear to be competing directly with each other—at least for the time being. For now they are focusing mainly on reducing healthcare costs by helping their own employees with better prevention and wellness, building on their own technical and business capabilities, and testing the waters with respect to healthcare in conditions they control (that is, their own clinics with their own providers and patients). But taken together, these ventures span much of the healthcare industry, from primary care to distribution to insurance, and they all share the goal of lowering costs.

Walgreens Boots Alliance–Microsoft

This unconventional alliance became public in January 2019 when drugstore chain Walgreens Boots Alliance announced it would partner with Microsoft in a multiyear research and development pact "to build health care solutions, improve health outcomes and lower the cost of care."

This partnership intends to shift the focus toward keeping patients healthy rather than treating them when they become sick. They will work to improve care in part by using patient information and the Walgreens store network to explore new ways of delivering healthcare while handing the tech giant hundreds of thousands of new users. Among other actions, the companies hope to boost prescription adherence, cut down on emergency room visits, and decrease hospital admissions.

The two companies plan to build "joint innovation centers" in key markets, while Walgreens will pilot test a dozen in-store "digital health corners" designed to show off and sell "select health care–related hardware and devices." In addition, Walgreens will move "the majority of the company's IT infrastructure" onto Microsoft Azure while also rolling out Microsoft 365 to the retailer's 380,000 employees around the world, according to a press release by Walgreens.

Walgreens and Microsoft are teaming up in response to potential competition from the aforementioned healthcare-related alliances. According to Stefano Pessina, executive vice chairman and chief executive officer of Walgreens Boots Alliance, "Our strategic partnership with Microsoft demonstrates our strong commitment to creating integrated, next-generation, digitally enabled health care delivery solutions for our customers, transforming our stores into modern neighborhood health destinations and expanding customer offerings."

As we said previously, it's too early to know how much disruption will take place, who will do the disrupting, or how fast it will happen. The bad news for incumbents is that the clock is already ticking. The good news is that, according to a study by PricewaterhouseCooper's global strategy consulting team (Strategy&), organizations facing disruption usually have longer to respond than they expect, and an effective response is typically available to them. Keep in mind that it took Amazon more than a decade to meaningfully disrupt traditional retail.

Although disruption can blindside industries (When was the last time you reached for an encyclopedia to find information? Rented a movie at a video store? Purchased film for a camera?), it is not axiomatic that disruption will lead to an industry's demise.

In hospitality, the rise of new, game-changing organizations such as VRBO and Airbnb has not hurt their more established hotel competitors—at least not yet. Hotels have experienced strong growth since 2008, even as the brokered, online vacation rental marketplace has been taking off. Travel across all demographic groups has increased, and the success of online vacation rental platforms has motivated the larger hotel chains like Wyndham, Marriott, InterContinental, Hilton, and others to raise their competitive game.

This book is a wake-up call for the healthcare industry to move toward consumer/patient–centric healthcare—where the consumer is in the center and in control, where helping people stay healthy is financially rewarded, and where healthcare is more accessible and affordable to all. We describe how healthcare leaders can position their organizations to disrupt themselves before someone else does (organizations such as Amazon, Apple, or Alphabet). The established healthcare business model is justifiably under assault, and we want to help healthcare leaders reframe it.

The question is not whether the healthcare industry *can* be disrupted. Nor is the question whether someone outside the industry *will* cause disruption. The question is how quickly outsiders will make meaningful disruptions to healthcare and whether today's existing organizations will play a role in charting the future. We do know this: adaptability and constant innovation to better serve consumers will be the keys to survival for medical providers.

RESHAPING HEALTHCARE FOR THE FUTURE

As we begin to consider ways to reshape healthcare for the future, it may be helpful to be aware of the different types of innovation, all of which are necessary for an organization's long-term success. Clayton Christensen, a professor at the Harvard Business School and author of *The Innovator's Prescription*, postulated three types of innovation:

» **Sustaining Innovation**: Innovation focused on improving existing products and services or replacing them with something better. This kind of innovation enables the incumbent to stay in business by not becoming obsolete, but does not help grow the business. The healthcare industry teems with examples: robotic and laser surgery, curing hepatitis C (albeit with very expensive drugs), mapping the genome, central scheduling, electronic health records, urgent care clinics, standardized care pathways, individual temperature controls in patient rooms, and electronic activity/exercise tracking.

» **Efficiency Innovation**: Innovation focused on improving existing processes. This type of innovation targets waste, excess cost, and lost revenue. If efficiencies are gained, efficiency innovation can increase the capacity of your business, but may not help you grow your business. Most of the process improvement activity over the years has been of this nature (examples include PDCA, CQI, TQM, Six Sigma, and Lean). Examples of efficiency innovation in healthcare include reduced waiting times, reduced procedure costs, reduced operating room turnaround times, improved safety, reduced readmission rates, and smoother handoff of patients from one unit to another.

» **Disruptive Innovation**: Innovation that creates new markets and/or value networks and eventually displaces established market-leading firms, products, and/or alliances. Innovation is disruptive when it enables a product or service to be simpler, more affordable, and easier to access, while, at least in healthcare, not sacrificing quality.

Disruptive innovation is a growth strategy for organizations and will be the primary focus of this book. Examples of disruptive innovation in healthcare include the following:

» The shift of care from hospitals to outpatient settings and eventually to the patient's home

» Primary care providers moving upmarket, thereby disrupting specialists

» Physician assistants performing a significant portion of the work primary care physicians are currently doing

» Providers and health coaches in a fixed fee arrangement who collaborate to reduce the need for medical treatments and hospitalizations

» Onsite 3-D printing of medications, supplies, medical equipment, and, eventually, body parts

» Direct employer-to-provider contracting that eliminates the need for insurance middlemen

» Mobile clinics that reduce the need for permanent ambulatory clinics

» Diagnostic equipment for at-home use

Here's an example how disruptive innovation works: If you think of a car dealership's service center as a hospital that has to be capable of treating every condition that comes in the door, then Jiffy Lube is an example of a clinic that specializes in one area, say orthopedics. The creators of Jiffy Lube looked at the dealership and asked something to the effect of "What high-volume services could we target and then design a convenient, customer-friendly, and inexpensive way to do the same thing?"

The answer was lube jobs and oil changes performed by inexpensive workers specifically trained to do those two tasks. This is much like an orthopedic clinic or surgery center that is easy to access and designed specifically for speed, lower cost, and high quality and is staffed by not only specialists but also other less expensive advance practice providers. This appeals to the physicians who own the clinics because they can charge less yet make more because they don't have to pay the 65 percent overhead that makes hospital care so expensive.

As management guru Peter Drucker said, "The greatest danger in times of turbulence is not the turbulence. It is to act with yesterday's logic."

While we encourage healthcare organizations to adopt disruptive innovation strategies and not act with yesterday's logic, the work of sustaining and efficiency innovation must continue. All types of innovation are needed now as much as ever before. In fact, it may be more important to get started with all types of innovation than to get confused over which type to employ. In our experience, efficiency innovation predominates in healthcare. While necessary, that will be insufficient as the industry faces intense consumer pressure for improved care and reduced costs.

Throughout this book, we will showcase and discuss the three types of innovation. All three are vital and necessary for a healthy, functional industry. But as far as we're concerned, the key is to upend healthcare as it currently exists.

Ultimately, we must empower consumers and patients, move them to an autonomous position, create a free-market environment for healthcare, take a proactive approach by keeping people healthy, and make necessary care less expensive and more accessible.

We will focus on what consumers and patients actually want and how healthcare leaders can meet those needs with the tools, technology, and information currently available. Our guiding principle will be putting consumers in the driver's seat of their own health, their own care, and their own health data.

Collectively, both of us have been involved in healthcare for over fifty years. We feel privileged to have had the opportunity to work with so many outstanding people. We are impressed by the passion, enthusiasm, determination, and caring that our coworkers and clients demonstrate by default—to the patients we all serve as well as to each other. Our experience has convinced us that healthcare is a calling rather than an occupation. People are drawn to health professions because they want to help people and enrich their lives. They want to heal individuals while achieving a bigger purpose for our society.

In the Preface we mentioned the lethal and nonlethal harm that unintentionally springs from the healthcare industry. We are in no way implying that any of the exceptional medical professionals deliberately intend to do harm of any sort. It is poorly designed work processes and systems, lack of standard work, and inadequate leadership that are at fault, rather than the dedicated professionals who toil within the system every day.

Having said that, the shockingly high number of fatalities and nonlethal harm that occur in healthcare every day are more than enough reason to dramatically reform the healthcare system. This book is intended to provide healthcare leaders with practical antidotes to cure our ailing system. We will start by examining four disruptive forces that will induce healthcare to change.

1

Why the Band-Aid Is about to Be Ripped off Traditional **Healthcare**

THE PRESSURE IS MOUNTING,
AND HEALTHCARE WILL BE
FORCED TO CHANGE.

MOVING FORWARD, THE CLUMSY
AND SLOW WILL EAT THE DUST
OF THE NIMBLE AND FAST.

The US economy has shifted to technology-based business, personal, and social conveniences. We have moved from bricks to clicks as consumers increasingly expect fast, sophisticated products and services that cater to their needs.

Walmart, Amazon, Facebook, and others have replaced the likes of Chevron, Ford, and Kodak as America's business stalwarts. Besides healthcare, we cannot think of any industry that has not been forced to adapt or many jobs that have not been impacted. We are living in an age of disruption—where new technologies and behavioral shifts are transforming the way we live. Disruptive forces are sweeping across the US economy. This disruption is real, it's big, it's happening faster, and it is here to stay.

"Disruptive innovation is not new; it's just that the pace of change is accelerating," observed our colleague, Phil Gibbs, PhD, president of The Disruption Lab in Nashville, Tennessee.

In this era of disruption, the most successful companies are those that measure their success through the lens of the consumer. The rise of new technologies, the proliferation of data, and stronger connectivity have made it possible to serve consumers in new ways that are more accessible, easier to use, and less expensive. This attracts fresh competitors who zero in on consumers' needs and use technology to remove superfluous steps, costs, and time. These disruptive companies are challenging the status quo and upending many traditional industries.

It's only natural that products and services are improving as consumer expectations evolve over time. Who doesn't want a better user experience, higher resolution, faster service, or better care? Consumers are demanding more choice and control than ever before, and increasing empowerment through technology is redefining what's important to consumers and further shaking up industries. Right now employers are increasingly driving disruption in healthcare. But we believe consumers will ultimately become the most important force for change in healthcare.

The convergence and blurring of previously distinct industries is also driving change. A company with a unique business model (such as Uber and Lyft) can enter an existing industry (transportation) with a better way to serve consumers and grab market share quickly. Traditional companies (such as taxis, in this case) must innovate or they will not survive. With respect to taxis, even while attempting to keep up by using newer and cleaner cars, better drivers, and becoming more customer focused, there is no guarantee they will survive.

Further, as industry boundaries become more porous, existing companies will face competitive threats from start-ups with new and game-changing business models as well as from formidable companies in previously unrelated industries (the way

Amazon, Apple, Alphabet, and other nonhealthcare organizations are attempting to disrupt healthcare).

The disruption we are beginning to experience in healthcare will render existing value propositions obsolete. But it also offers vast opportunities for growth to those able to see the potential upside and who are willing to seize it. The future belongs to those who can think differently to engage consumers in creative ways, find solutions to problems, and deliver increasing value.

What are the major disruptive forces that will impact healthcare?

We begin by discussing the age wave that is hitting US shores. Demographic changes within our population will necessitate significant change for medical providers.

We then highlight a few organizations that are changing the competitive landscape by overturning existing business models and boundaries. We previously mentioned the likes of Amazon, Apple, Alphabet, and Walgreens, but what about other organizations that are disrupting existing business models in healthcare? What might we learn from their disruptive forces? We highlight companies in different industries that are taking interesting and creative approaches to reining in health costs. These are large employers who are proactively looking at the health of their employees and demanding more from healthcare.

We then discuss savvy medical providers who have risen to the challenge to meet employer needs and end with summaries of a few key disruptive technologies that will impact healthcare.

DISRUPTIVE FORCE #1
POPULATION AGE WAVE

In a concept first identified in 1990 by Ken Dychtwald in a book titled *The Age Wave*, the United States is in the midst of an age boom. Every day, more than 10,000 Americans turn sixty-five, and in general, those over age fifty are expected to live longer than any previous generation. The Census Bureau projects the country's elderly population will double to 88 million by 2050, taking the number of people sixty-five and older to 26 percent.

In many respects having more time with our elders is a blessing. We'll have more time to engage with them, learn with them, love them, and expand our memories of them to comfort us when they are gone. However, as our population ages, Dychtwald believes "the epicenter of consumer activity will shift from a focus on youth to the needs, challenges, and aspirations of maturing consumers."

According to Dychtwald, the age wave is putting unprecedented pressure on families, communities, and governments as multiplying numbers of older adults strain healthcare and eldercare. In fact, an estimated ten to twelve million elderly citizens need some form of health-related help at any given time.

Compounding the impact of the aging baby boom generation is our country's increasing life expectancy. Thanks to advances in public health, nutrition management, and medical science, life expectancy in the US has steadily increased throughout the twentieth century—rising from 47 years in 1900 to 78.6 years in 2017. However, while we've managed to prolong life-span, we've lagged far behind in extending people's health span.

Our modern healthcare system is incompetent at preventing and treating the complex and intertwined conditions of later life. According to HuffPost, Alzheimer's and related dementias now afflict half the people over eighty-five. Unless there is a breakthrough, its sufferers are anticipated to grow from 5+ million today to 15+ million as the boomers age, with its cumulative costs soaring to $20 trillion by 2050.

Unfortunately, our medical priorities are not aligned with this reality. For every dollar currently spent on Alzheimer's care, less than half a cent is being spent on research for prevention. In addition, our doctors are not ready for the increased need for eldercare. The US has more than 50,000 pediatricians, but fewer than 5,000 geriatricians. Only eight of the country's 145 academic medical centers have full geriatrics departments, and 97 percent of US medical students don't take a single course in geriatrics.

With respect to health insurance, members of the baby boom generation are moving from commercial insurance to Medicare at the rate of 10,000 per day. AARP suggests this will happen every year going forward until 2030.

As a bit of background, the modern healthcare system is built on cross-subsidy. Generally speaking, commercial health insurers like Blue Cross Blue Shield, Aetna, and Humana pay the highest level of reimbursement to hospitals and medical providers. Medicare pays less than these commercial insurers, while Medicaid reimburses at even lower levels.

So, as 3.65 million baby boomers per year retire and move to Medicare, what was once higher margin care for patients with commercial insurance is rapidly eroding into lower margin care. In the past, as Medicare and Medicaid rolls increased, medical providers and pharmaceutical companies simply raised prices to cover their costs and provide margin. In other words, people with commercial insurance subsidized those on Medicare and Medicaid. However, annual double-digit price increases for those with commercial insurance are becoming increasingly difficult as employers push back.

Moving forward, medical providers are going to have to learn how to provide high-quality, convenient, customer-centric care much cheaper than they are now, or they will not survive.

DISRUPTIVE FORCE #2
FRUSTRATED EMPLOYERS WHO
HAVE HAD ENOUGH

Employers in various industries are beginning to disrupt healthcare by taking interesting and creative approaches to the way they provide health coverage for their employees. Although

Amazon, Apple, and Google are receiving the most attention, you would be mistaken if you think they are the only companies trying new ways to rein in health costs. In fact, business coalitions and Chambers of Commerce around the country are in full-throated revolt with the healthcare industry about sustained, unreasonable price increases.

"People don't actually want to think about their own health and don't take action until they are sick. Yet employers are very motivated to get their employees healthy, since they bear most of the burden of their health care costs," said Clayton Christensen in *The Innovator's Prescription: A Disruptive Solution for Health Care.*

Every employer is doing something to control their healthcare costs, and the number and variety of organizations that are beginning to fundamentally change how they view the health of their workforce as well as the provision of healthcare to them might surprise you.

US corporations help pay for healthcare for more than 170 million Americans. These employers spent an estimated $738 billion on health benefits in 2018, a figure that has been rising about 5 percent annually in recent years.

Largely due to frustration with incessantly rising costs, some large companies are discarding long-held practices and adopting a do-it-yourself approach. We're not talking about the popular routes of squeezing extra discounts from providers and insurers, or of having employees bear more of the rising costs through high-deductible plans. Instead, innovative companies are moving toward empowering staff by providing support and assistance to help them make better decisions for themselves and their families regarding health and healthcare. These organizations have turned to independent services to help staff navigate the fragmented and confusing healthcare marketplace. Some have even gone beyond healthcare to help employees in other related areas such as improving financial literacy.

The underlying precept for these organizations is that the focus should be on employee health and wellness. They also believe employees should not feel alone, confused, or overwhelmed when it comes to understanding and choosing healthcare for themselves or loved ones. In addition, a few companies have partnered directly with medical providers to deliver services to their staff and their family members, bypassing traditional health insurance plans altogether.

Here we highlight a few companies who have taken novel approaches regarding the health and healthcare of their employees. This is not intended to be a comprehensive accounting of all innovative employers, but rather to give a sense for what forward-thinking organizations in different industries are doing to transform healthcare and to reduce healthcare spending.

It is our belief that the increasingly widespread refusal by employers to pay the never-ending price increases and to create alternative arrangements have been the matches that started the fire of innovative disruption in healthcare.

Walmart

Yes, Walmart uses its size (2.4 million employees, not including their families) and influence to negotiate with health insurers and providers for the best rates and options for their associates. But they have also been at the forefront of efforts to direct staff to specific providers to receive medical care, even if it means paying their travel to out-of-state hospitals.

In 2013 Walmart launched an innovative Centers of Excellence (COE) program that covered all expenses, including travel, for costly, complicated heart and spine surgeries at six reputable healthcare centers. The following year, Walmart expanded the program to include knee and hip replacement surgeries and, in 2015, added breast, lung, and colorectal cancer care. To help its employees with medical problems not yet included within the COE, Walmart uses services such as HealthCompare and DirectHealth to provide personalized guidance for their associates in finding appropriate, affordable healthcare.

In starting its COE program, Walmart was striving for better surgical results and cost savings, which they've achieved. But they also realized big improvements in care and cost savings from avoiding procedures that shouldn't be done in the first place. Walmart's COE includes these six medical providers, as indicated on the map below:

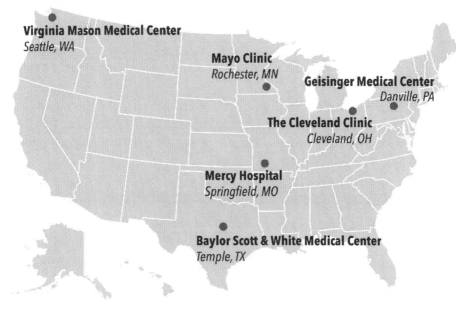

Virginia Mason Medical Center
Seattle, WA

Mayo Clinic
Rochester, MN

Geisinger Medical Center
Danville, PA

The Cleveland Clinic
Cleveland, OH

Mercy Hospital
Springfield, MO

Baylor Scott & White Medical Center
Temple, TX

The six medical providers under Walmart's
Centers of Excellence program.

Beyond what they are doing for associates, Walmart has an ambitious vision regarding health and healthcare, including potentially taking on the risk for a large patient population. They are in early talks with Humana about strengthening their existing partnership, and possibly acquiring the insurer. Such a move could reshape healthcare in ways even the stoutest competitor would have trouble matching. Walmart had previously approached online pharmacy start-up PillPack, but was thwarted by Amazon who subsequently purchased the innovative pharmacy.

As the country's largest private employer and one of the country's largest retailers, Walmart recognizes the enormous potential it has to make a meaningful difference and has strived to make healthcare and healthier food more affordable and accessible for consumers. Over the years, Walmart has ramped up its health offerings, from pharmacy to care delivery, all with a focus on affordability. Most notably, this includes a list of prescription drugs Walmart sells for $4 through its 4,500 pharmacies, with no insurance required. According to the company, this service has saved consumers more than $3 billion since it was launched over a decade ago.

Walmart also offers access to medical and vision care. They have 2,900 vision centers, have rolled out primary care clinics that operate inside a smaller number of Walmart stores, and in 2017 began offering lab testing services in some Florida and Texas locations.

Walmart has also focused on preventive care and overall well-being through in-store events, online education, and an expanded assortment of products and services available both in-store and online. To bring transparency and simplicity to the changing health insurance market, Walmart partnered with DirectHealth.com to launch *Healthcare Begins Here*, an in-store program to educate consumers on health insurance options. This provides a resource that brings Walmart customers unprecedented access to health insurance information and enrollment support.

Comcast

Perhaps not a name most people would associate with healthcare innovation, Comcast has set itself apart by its willingness to tackle its medical costs directly rather than relying on others.

To lower costs while providing excellent care for over 150,000 staff (not including their families), Comcast uses a variety of strategies. Comcast employees with company coverage are encouraged to initially go to Accolade—an on-demand, personalized advocacy and population health solution that uses independent health navigators to help people make the best decisions about their healthcare, as well as to connect them to the resources they need. Accolade's phone number even appears on the back of employee insurance cards.

Accolade navigators routinely help find medical providers, guide employees through complicated medical decisions, find the most affordable care options, manage symptoms after surgery, and help employees understand benefits for which they qualify.

Comcast employees also have access to Grand Rounds, a company that connects patients with local and remote specialty physicians. For Comcast employees, Grand Rounds is often used to provide a second opinion if their family physician recommends a complicated or costly procedure. In complicated cases, Grand Rounds has served as a check on decisions or recommendations made by the network or insurer.

In addition to helping employees stay physically healthy, the next frontier for Comcast was the financial literacy and well-being of its employees, many of whom live paycheck to paycheck and struggle to afford small copayments toward provider visits. Previously, employees who ran into financial trouble had no independent source of information.

After talking to many vendors, Comcast was unable to find a financial services firm that would help employees without trying to sell products or earn money on commissions. So Comcast created and invested in a new company called Brightside, an online platform to reduce employee financial stress. The underlying thinking is that employees who are less worried about their finances will be happier and more engaged and thus less likely to miss work or suffer from health problems.

It's too early to know for certain what impact this program is having, but as far as we're concerned, increasing people's financial literacy should command our attention because it impacts many facets of our lives, including healthcare, education, retirement, and general well-being.

General Motors

With a goal of lowering costs and improving care, GM signed a direct contract with Detroit-based Henry Ford Health System to provide a wide range of healthcare services for its 24,000 salaried employees and their dependents in Southeast Michigan. This agreement covers everything from routine doctor visits to surgical procedures and includes a number of consumer-friendly functions such as a concierge line for GM employees to make appointments and get directions; telehealth options for employees to interact with doctors by phone, video chat, or computer/smartphone app; and same-day appointments for primary care doctors and appointments with specialists within ten days.

This approach upends traditional health-benefits arrangements in which companies hire insurers for access to a broader network of healthcare providers. In those cases, insurers negotiate the prices with hospitals, doctors, and other providers, and employers seldom have access to the terms that govern their medical costs. By signing a contract directly with one healthcare provider—as several other large, self-insured companies have done—GM believes it can offer a plan that costs employees less while also promising high-quality care and special customer-service perks.

Under the five-year contract, Henry Ford must meet an annual financial budget and will be held accountable for hitting targets on nineteen agreed-upon metrics, including customer service, preventive care, quality, ER visits, and utilization of a wide range of services. This is a contracting paradigm that moves away from fee-for-service medicine and encourages quality and value-based care. If Henry Ford remains under the total annual cost terms and hits the other metrics, the system will split the savings with GM. But if the targets are not reached, Henry Ford could lose money.

According to the National Business Group on Health (NBGH), approximately 3 percent of self-insured companies nationally have some form of direct contracts with providers. NBGH also found that 11 percent of employers indicated they plan to pursue direct contracts with healthcare providers in 2019. However, other sources predict even faster adoption of centers of excellence and direct contracting. Investment bank Leerink Partners reports that "nearly 80 percent of large employers have said they will use COEs by 2019, while 22 percent expect to directly contract with health systems."

We believe these percentages will increase exponentially in the ensuing years. GM is just the latest in a growing list of high-profile employers—including Cisco, Disney, General Electric, Intel, and Lowe's—that are choosing to negotiate their own terms directly with healthcare providers. Others will certainly follow as a way to reduce healthcare costs, improve service, and shrink the role of health insurance middlemen.

Like the other large employers with direct-to-provider arrangements, an insurer will still play a role in GM's relationship with Henry Ford Health System. Blue Cross Blue Shield of Michigan will manage claims processing and other functions.

Boeing

Boeing has realized the benefits from direct-to-provider plans with health systems. Boeing began its direct contracting in 2015 and now has such setups in its multiple US locations. In negotiating its direct partner contracts, Boeing placed a high priority on access and convenience for its employees.

Primary care appointments for acute conditions are available the same day and within seventy-two hours for any condition. The wait for a specialist appointment can be no longer than ten days. In addition, Boeing's contracts include extended hours, a dedicated phone line with care navigators, an employee website, and mobile apps. Boeing is also emphasizing greater attention to preventive and maintenance care.

By applying the same commitment to better quality, increased reliability, and lower costs to healthcare as it does to building aircraft, Boeing is saving money for itself and employees while improving health services, enhancing employee health, and creating a more positive experience for employees. Boeing, who spends approximately $2.5 billion annually on healthcare for more than 480,000 US workers, their dependents, and retirees, is striving to save $350 to $1,000 per person per year on monthly payments.

In one of its markets, Boeing has taken an even more ambitious tact to direct contracting by having the healthcare provider manage nearly all of the care of enrolled employees and assume the risks traditionally born by insurance companies. Mercy Health Alliance, the accountable care organization Boeing contracted directly with in St. Louis, pledged to cut the average per family healthcare costs by more than half—from $15,849 to $6,000 per year—by focusing on prevention and maintenance care.

While Boeing made an early attempt to create a consumer-centric retail market where its employees had a broad range of coverage options, other large organizations have already done so for their retiree benefits. These include Walgreens, CVS, and IBM. Although participation in consumer-provider retail markets is currently small, it is highly likely this trend will increase as employers increasingly come to see this as a compelling way to control costs, improve care, and reduce administrative burdens.

Interestingly, smaller employers and individual consumers may come to rely on a pair of unlikely sources for access to consumer-centric retail markets—Sam's Club and Costco. Both membership-driven price clubs have partnered with Aetna to offer their respective plans, which enable small employers to offer affordable health coverage to their employees (Sam's Club) and for individuals to purchase coverage in the growing retail market for health services (Costco).

By attempting to create consumer-centric retail markets, Boeing, Walmart, and others are generating conditions long proven to bring down prices while improving quality: empowering and incenting consumers to seek value, stimulating competition among healthcare providers, and increasing the supply of medical care.

Once consumer-centric retail markets take hold and become mainstream, the consequences will be profound. Health insurers will become obsolete, and a robust retail market for individual health plans where consumers contract directly with providers, who are competing for consumer business, will supersede the group health insurance that most people are familiar with. As consumer-centric retail markets take hold, the cost of medical care will dramatically decline as tens of millions of consumers search for the best deal they can get for themselves and their families!

DISRUPTIVE FORCE #3
SAVVY COMPETITORS WHO VIEW
HEALTHCARE AS A BUSINESS

If the first two threats to medical providers are aging baby boomers and employers who are demanding more from the healthcare industry, the third threat is innovative medical providers who are already meeting that need by fundamentally changing how they view staff wellness and deliver care to those employees.

These innovative healthcare companies are helping employers to empower their staff by focusing on prevention and helping employees make better decisions for themselves and their families regarding health and healthcare.

They are redirecting care to the most appropriate level, often forgoing expensive procedures in place of therapies and other less costly interventions. They have partnered directly with employers to provide services to their employees and family members, bypassing traditional health insurance plans altogether. They are upending medical delivery and providing care with the same level of clinical quality and outcomes at 40 to 50 percent of the cost of traditional medical providers. And the patients themselves are more satisfied. These are the emerging competitors (and disruptive threats) for all medical providers, regardless of their physical location.

Employers Centers of Excellence Network

The Pacific Business Group on Health is a nonprofit, employer-led organization that represents public and employer healthcare purchasers. Health Design Plus (HDP) is a third-party administrator with expertise in the development and management of travel surgery programs. Inspired by several pioneering employers (like Walmart) who wanted to provide employees access to affordable, high-quality medical care, these organizations launched the Employers Centers of Excellence Network (ECEN) to help self-insured employers provide their employees with high-quality surgical care for certain high-cost procedures.

ECEN began in 2014 with total joint replacement, then added spinal surgery, and in 2018 began providing bariatric surgery at carefully selected centers of excellence (COEs) around the country. ECEN provides employees of participating companies with 100 percent coverage for all travel and medical expenses at the COEs. Participating employers benefit from the quality assurance of the ECEN's rigorous COE selection process and the financial savings from paying competitive, preset rates for bundled care negotiated between participating hospitals and HDP.

ECEN's Centers of Excellence includes the seven medical providers, as indicated on the map below:

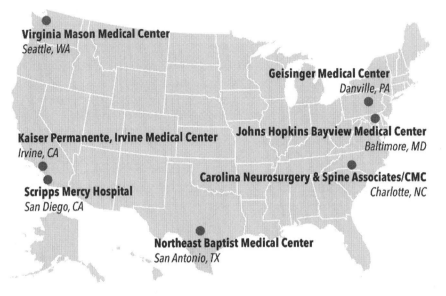

The seven medical providers that are part of ECEN's Centers of Excellence program.

Source data for this graphic was used with permission of ECEN.

Even when factoring in travel expenses and waived copays, ECEN's negotiated bundled payments for surgical procedures performed at the COEs cost considerably less than what members currently pay for these services locally. The value proposition improves even more because the participating COEs produce quality outcomes that reduce costly infections, surgical revisions, and readmissions. Even more cost mitigation comes from avoiding unnecessary procedures, with COEs using evidence-based medicine to determine surgical appropriateness.

Since its inception in 2014, the program has led to lower patient out-of-pocket costs, improved patient outcomes and satisfaction, reduced costs for employers, as well as improved processes and efficiencies beyond the COE program for participating hospitals. The program has also prevented a large number of unnecessary surgical procedures, instead using activity-based therapies, injections for pain, physical therapy, and weight loss as more appropriate treatments.

The need for such treatment diversions is supported by a RAND Corporation study, which found that about 17 percent of high-cost emergency department (ED) visits could be diverted to a lower-cost, convenient care location such as urgent care centers or retail clinics, and that every 1 percent of high-cost care diverted from the ED to urgent care would account for $1 billion in savings.

Centers of excellence programs are proving to be worth the investment because they increase value for patients, purchasers, and hospitals by improving patient outcomes and satisfaction, decreasing costs for patients and employers, and increasing volumes for the participating COE health systems. Such centers of excellence are part of broader travel medicine programs that, as we will address later, are even moving internationally.

Not all centers of excellence are created equal. Branded centers of excellence (COEs) have become more common as hospitals attempt to highlight the quality of clinical services aimed at treating specific ailments such as joint replacement surgery, bariatric surgery, and stroke care, among others. These organizations have adopted or created specific and measurable criteria that the program and physicians must meet to be deemed a COE.

The criteria typically include program infrastructure, surgeon and hospital experience levels, procedure volumes, clinical quality, and patient outcomes. Insurers have begun to establish similar criteria for their own COE designations, and the Joint Commission has also begun to certify institutions in care for specific diseases.

Unlike the ECEN Centers of Excellence or those of Walmart, the rigor of standards varies across self-designated COEs, and some are little more than marketing strategies. What sets the

ECEN and Walmart apart are uniform and rigorous standards for clinical quality along with free-market pricing. Genuine centers of excellence consist of physicians (including specialists and surgeons) and healthcare facilities who offer up-front, transparent, bundled pricing. These COEs also help consumers save money by preventing a large number of unnecessary surgical procedures.

At-Risk Providers Focus on Personalized Wellness and Cost Transparency

What if a new healthcare organization came into town and sold a local hospital's larger payers on a new model that is fully at risk, significantly less costly, more accessible, with quality just as good? What if they really knew how to manage employee populations in such a way that there were 40 percent fewer hospitalizations and the overall cost was reduced by 20 percent? How threatening would that be to the status quo, fee-for-service hospital? The truth of the matter is that such companies already exist.

Two examples are Paladina Health and Iora Health. Dedicated care teams and price transparency are at the heart of these medical providers' approach to patient wellness. Their focus is on providing the right care for patients rather than what insurance companies will reimburse for.

To accomplish this, both organizations invested heavily in increasing primary care physicians (PCPs) and having them take on some of the work performed by specialists (by hiring specialists as consultants to the PCPs), moving portions of primary care work to health coaches to keep consumers healthy and out of the hospitals in the first place, and, where appropriate, moving some of the care to the patient by helping them change unhealthy behaviors.

Health coaches work with patients and intervene the moment trouble arises, especially with chronic care patients whose costliest problem is noncompliance. These coaches engage patients in new ways, including smoking cessation clinics, helping diabetic patients shop for food, teaching Zumba classes, training patients to monitor blood pressure and insulin levels, and so forth. This moving of work to different levels, from doctors to health coaches and from health coaches to patients, saves money.

The capitated payment system, however, was the real difference. Under the been-around-far-too-long fee-for-service models, providers need a high volume of patient visits and procedures in order to make money. Under a capitation system, Paladina and Iora make money only if their patients stay healthy and require fewer tests and procedures. This completely different business model is focused on value, relationships, outcomes, and the long game.

Patients are truly the focus with Paladina and Iora. Patients have access to better medical service through next-day appointments, telemedicine, longer visits, emails with providers, and more integrated care that includes a doctor, nurse, and health coach working with the patient to set goals—empowering patients to be more active in their care. Further, a stratified approach to primary care (that is, low need, rising need, chronic care) ensures patients receive the right amount of care and attention.

By placing consumers' health at the center of their business model, Iora and Paladina have not just improved patients' health, they've also lowered costs significantly. For example, by 2017, seven years after launching, Iora Health had reduced hospitalizations for its members by 40 percent and cut total healthcare spending by 15 percent to 20 percent. Their patient retention rate was 98 percent, and their Net Promoter Score among patients was in the 90s (this is a measure of how willing someone is to recommend an organization's products and services to others, which correlates strongly with growth). Further, some 90 percent of patients had their blood pressure under control, compared with an average of 60 percent across the industry. Employee attrition was only 2.5 percent.

What Iora and Paladina have demonstrated is that it is not all that expensive to provide care—unless the care is given in a hospital, where 60 to 65 percent of the expense is fixed cost (overhead).

Iora Health was started in 2010 by Rushika Fernandopulle, an entrepreneur and Harvard-trained physician. He saw several things that bothered him about the current healthcare system, including the widespread fee-for-service payment system that incented performing unneeded tests and procedures, the fact that so little (only 4 to 5%) of the total cost of care was spent on primary care, and healthcare IT platforms that did everything except support patient care delivery.

Because primary care accounted for such a small percentage of the total cost of care, he felt the system was backward—sick care instead of helping people stay healthy. Fernandopulle instituted a fully capitated payment system focused on primary care that required no fees, no coinsurance, and no copays. His goal was not just to deliver better healthcare, but also to empower patients to change their behavior.

Iora charged employers a flat monthly fee per member that was twice their historical spend on primary care, money that has proven to be easily recouped by keeping people out of the hospital. He hired four health coaches for every primary care physician and made them a critical component of patient care.

Iora initially opened four offices, each with a self-insured employer or union benefits manager as its chief insurance partner. They selected sites from different parts of the country including New Hampshire (Dartmouth College), Las Vegas (Culinary Health Fund), Brooklyn (Freelancers Union), and Dorchester, Massachusetts (New England Carpenters Benefit Funds). They have grown significantly since their inception, demonstrating that the model works across the country. In June 2018, Iora secured $100 million in funding to support their growth and technology platform. Their model works and is proving to be a major disruptor. Status quo hospitals beware.

Ambulatory Surgery Centers

From their humble beginnings in the early 1970s, ambulatory surgery centers (ASCs) offer a low-cost, high-quality alternative for many surgical procedures and are part of a trend toward surgical procedures being performed outside hospital operating rooms. Across the United States, ASCs are increasing in both number and surgical volume—there are presently 5,480 Medicare-certified ASCs (compared to 5,564 registered hospitals), and in 2017 more than 20 million Americans entrusted ASCs for outpatient surgical procedures and treatments ranging from cataract surgery to total joint replacement.

The map below shows the number of Medicare-certified ambulatory surgery centers in each state.

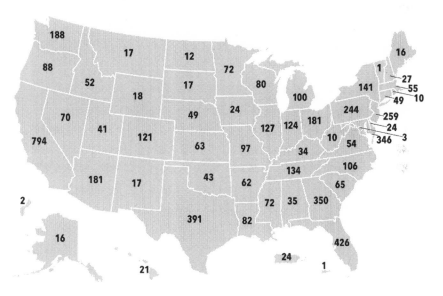

Number of Medicare-certified ambulatory surgical centers, by state.

Source data for this graphic was used with permission of the Ambulatory Surgical Center Association.

ASCs have been a focus of debate regarding reimbursement, patient safety, as well as surgical productivity and efficiency. But the surgeons, anesthesiologists, nurses, and other health professionals who practice in ASCs have the same education, training, and talent as their peers who work exclusively in hospitals, and they care just as much about their patients. The reasons behind the growing demand for outpatient surgeries encompass many characteristics consumers want in healthcare, including convenience, lower cost, better efficiency and dependability, state-of-the-art medical equipment, and high-quality care with good clinical outcomes.

Because our healthcare system is risk averse, new procedures move into the ASC setting only after the medical community is convinced that the surgical technique, anesthesia, pain control, and recovery time associated with these outpatient procedures support the same outcomes as when those procedures are performed in the hospital. Further, ASCs have long supported meaningful healthcare quality reporting and continue to improve systems that help patients make informed decisions.

As we'll argue throughout this book, patients deserve better access to data on the safety, quality, and cost of the care they are to receive, regardless of what the procedure is or where it takes place.

According to Dr. James Lozada, "ASCs also have a demonstrated record of providing real value to patients. The cost of procedures performed in surgery centers are nearly always less than the same procedures performed in hospital outpatient departments. For example, the ASC costs for Medicare beneficiaries are approximately 50% less than hospital outpatient departments. In addition, a review of commercial claims data found that US health care costs are reduced by more than $38 billion per year due to the availability of ASCs as an appropriate setting for care. Further, over $5 billion of those savings directly benefit patients through lower deductible and coinsurance payments."

Several experts have pointed out the risks to having surgery in outpatient settings. The fact is that any surgery carries risk, no matter where the procedure is done. The vast majority of operations performed in ambulatory surgery centers go off without a hitch. Adverse medical events are rare and occur across all sites of care, including hospitals. Further, there is no empirical evidence suggesting ambulatory surgery centers pose any more risk to patients than hospitals. The people who practice in ASCs are the same as those who practice in hospitals—healthcare professionals dedicated to helping patients.

Here's one example. Founded in 1997, the Surgery Center of Oklahoma (SCO) is one of the many ambulatory surgery centers in the US. They have a 32,535-square-foot, state-of-the-art, multispecialty facility in Oklahoma City, which is owned and operated by over fifty of the top surgeons and anesthesiologists in central Oklahoma. The SCO is accredited by the Accreditation Association for Ambulatory Health Care; they provide outpatient adult and pediatric surgeries; and their specialists perform more than 6,000 surgeries each year.

Transparent, direct package pricing is at the heart of the Surgery Center of Oklahoma's mission, vision, and values, and ensures that all patients know exactly what the cost of the service will be up front. The pricing outlined on the SCO website is not a teaser or a bait-and-switch. It is the actual price consumers will pay. They can offer these prices because they are completely physician-owned and managed. They also control every aspect of the facility from real estate costs to the most efficient use of staff, to the elimination of wasteful operating room practices that are prevalent in many hospitals.

The staff at the Surgery Center of Oklahoma understand that patients are paying more and more out of pocket, and they are committed to providing the best quality care at the lowest possible price.

Not only do many uninsured or underinsured American patients take advantage of SCO's cash pricing, but many Canadians have traveled there to receive care. SCO's focus has expanded to working with self-funded employers to offer high-value care to their employees. Increasingly, self-funded health plans are taking advantage of the SCO's transparent pricing model and realizing significant savings to their employee health plans.

Free Market Medical Association

The free-market movement in healthcare is gaining steam because of providers, patients, and self-funded employers who believe changing the way people purchase healthcare services is necessary, and that seeking out value-driven healthcare providers is important.

By matching willing buyers with willing sellers of healthcare services, the Free Market Medical Association (FMMA) plays the same third-party broker role for healthcare that Uber and Lyft play for transportation or that Airbnb and VRBO play for lodging. With the goal of uniting and strengthening the benefits of free-market healthcare, FMMA helps connect

> » Patients (insured or uninsured) who are looking to find fair pricing for healthcare,

> » Free-market physicians (including specialists and surgeons) and healthcare facilities who offer up-front, transparent, bundled pricing,

> » Employers who want to reduce healthcare spending and budget appropriately while increasing or maintaining health benefits for their staff, and

> » Patient advocates who are helping make everything work.

FMMA's goal is to unite and strengthen the benefits of free-market healthcare with the mission to unite all of the islands of excellence in healthcare and accelerate the speed and growth of the free-market healthcare revolution.

FMMA members are able to connect with other like-minded individuals who are motivated to change the healthcare landscape. In addition to providing networking opportunities, FMMA educates physicians, facilities, self-funded businesses, patients, third-party administrators, and other healthcare service vendors in how to further the movement. FMMA members and supporters include long-standing free-market warriors, those who are just learning about the movement, and everyone in between.

Due to the wildly varying definitions of transparency and free market in the healthcare industry (many of which are neither free market nor transparent), FMMA has designated three pillars as the foundation of the association. FMMA members are asked to always abide by these pillars, using ethics and transparency in all areas of their businesses. As far as FMMA is concerned, the free market only works when there is freedom of choice that includes an informed, willing buyer and a willing seller with transparent pricing.

FMMA's three pillars include price, value, and equality.

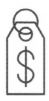

PRICE

PRICE is not a product. Care is the product.

Selling access to pricing is anti-free market

Discount brokers who get paid by selling "savings" are not transparent.

VALUE

VALUE is established when the buyer and seller agree on a fully disclosed, mutually beneficial price for care.

If a vendor adds or changes that price in any way, those amounts should be truthfully disclosed.

EQUALITY

Price EQUALITY is the basis of a free market

Cash is king.

Any willing cash buyer should be offered the same price regardless of any factor.

PRICE

Health plans have been forced to rely on PPOs/networks, or specialty discount vendors, to give them access to a percentage off "billed charges" contracts in an effort to reduce truly outrageous charges. This system has done nothing to curb the rising cost of care and has, instead, contributed to the increase. By selling access to a discounted price, it is highly beneficial to the establishment if the charges are excessive.

Percentage-based payment models incent price gouging and pricing games. Selling access to a discount where you benefit from the price being high puts you at odds with the best interests of the buyers and sellers of healthcare.

Examples of scenarios where the vendor wins when healthcare costs go up are these:

» Percentage of savings

» Percentage of claims

» Percentage of premium

VALUE

In an open free market, consumers can readily access the information to choose healthcare providers based on value. Value is based on price *and* quality. A consumer cannot determine the value of the purchasing choices they make without price honesty.

Our current healthcare system employs a magician's bag full of tricks to hide the real price from the buyer. Costs will never decrease until consumers can make fully educated, value-based decisions about their care.

Hiding, modifying, or tampering with the true price for any reason is anti–free market. If facilitation of the service is requested, these facilitators and vendors should disclose their fees up front, openly, and honestly.

EQUALITY

In an open and honest free market, cash is always king. Enhanced discounts for guaranteed bodies through the door increases costs for patients based on factors they cannot control such as one insurance versus another. These are all symptoms of a broken system.

In a free-market system, a competitive price can be knowable, publishable, and complete regardless of who the patient is and the patient's insurance coverage.

Local chapters of FMMA function as a leg of the national association, promoting the ideals and goals at a local level. These local chapters not only provide support and encouragement to each other, but also resources that can drastically change the local landscape of the medical marketplace.

FMMA was founded on a true belief in transparency and a genuine desire to change how employers and participants view and purchase healthcare. FMMA has helped self-funded employers as well as countless individual consumers save millions of dollars, and they continuously strive to help them partner with free-market providers to improve health and lower healthcare costs.

We believe an increasing number of employers will join companies such as Walmart, Boeing, Lowe's, McKesson, and JetBlue by becoming part of a center of excellence network, directing employees to free-market medical providers and ambulatory surgical centers, and participating in travel medicine within the United States. We also believe such programs will expand beyond our shores to encompass medical providers around the world.

Medical Tourism

Given a choice, many Americans would view obtaining their healthcare outside of the United States unfavorably. This is not only due to the greater distance, but also to questions regarding the quality and medical expertise available elsewhere.

Interestingly, the latter is similar to what many established companies initially thought about disruptive upstarts (such as Blockbuster about Netflix, book sellers and retailers about Amazon, and the US steel industry about foreign competitors).

During the 2009–2010 time period, Aaron delivered a presentation titled "The Future of Healthcare" to audiences across the country. He cited a 2008 report that predicted the number of US tourists traveling out of the country for medical care could reach as high as 24 million by 2017. The actual number is currently in the 2.6 to 3.4 million range, with the bulk of those trips made by patients in the Southwestern US traveling to Mexico for low-cost, high-value medical and dental care.

Medical tourism has failed to live up to the original hype for several reasons. Currently, few health insurers will pay for such travel or invest in the concept. This is due to the difficulty of estimating the risk associated with care in foreign countries. A second reason is uncertainty regarding service recovery and the lack of recourse if something goes wrong in a foreign country.

Other countries don't have the same kinds of laws and legal protections afforded to citizens in the United States. We acknowledge these concerns as valid but believe they will become less of an issue as employers seeking the most affordable, high-quality care begin paying for employee healthcare services directly to medical providers. We also believe the issues around service recovery and legal protections in foreign countries will be resolved.

Although medical tourism numbers are not coming close to the lofty numbers predicted by the prognosticators in 2008, we believe the phenomenon of medical tourism will grow as employers and individual consumers facing higher deductible coverage or no coverage at all seek medical procedures at a lower cost. The emergence of and publicity around foreign medical providers delivering high-quality, low-cost care will also accelerate medical tourism, which offers the possibility of worldwide access to preventive/wellness services as well as acute care at highly competitive prices with equal or better clinical quality and outcomes.

One such wake-up call for US medical providers comes from Bangalore, India, where heart surgeons at Narayana Health perform up to 37 daily heart surgeries on adults and children at an average cost of $1,800. That translates to approximately 900 procedures a month (about what most US academic medical centers perform in a year) at 2 percent of the $90,000 average cost for heart surgery in the United States. The entire surgical experience is state-of-the-art, and beyond what is available almost anywhere else in the world.

And with respect to quality, patient outcomes are among the best in the world. The success at Narayana Health results from a combination of high-volume, advanced technology, and a focus on people and performance. But that's not enough. Driven by a deep desire to make healthcare affordable to all people in India— most of the patients do not even have health insurance—the physicians and staff at Narayana Health are working to reduce their cost even more.

Here's how medical tourism works in real life. A middle-aged woman in the United States was diagnosed with Dupuytren's (a gradual thickening and tightening of tissue under the skin in the hands) and Ledderhose disease (a rare condition that causes connective tissue to build up and create hard lumps on the bottoms of the feet). The pain in her feet was interfering with everyday activities as well as inhibiting her ability to perform her professional duties.

After extensive research, she chose to be treated at the Cyberknife Center in Hamburg, Germany, with radiation therapy in all four limbs. The results were excellent, and the cost was significantly less than comparable treatments in the US, even factoring in return trips to Germany for follow-up exams and treatments. Her quality of life and activity level are very good, and she is grateful to have her life back.

In Central America and South America, the International Hospital Management Corporation (IHMC, with headquarters in the Dallas/Fort Worth area) operates several healthcare facilities. Each hospital utilizes best practices from throughout the region, is modeled after successful facilities in the United States, and provides a full range of surgical, emergency, and diagnostic services.

IHMC's flagship hospital—Hospital CIMA San José in Costa Rica—opened in 2000 and has medical and surgical patient units, an intensive care unit, and a neonatal intensive care unit. Hospital CIMA San José is fully accredited by the Joint Commission International, meeting the organization's international standards for quality and patient safety. The hospital has also received Global Quality Certification from the Latin American Quality Institute.

When founded in 1992, IHMC's sole focus was to provide the kind of high-quality healthcare that had long prompted residents of those countries to travel to the United States for treatment. Over the years, they have found themselves playing host to a steady increase of North American residents who are crossing borders in search of affordable, high-quality care. Although their main customers are residents in the countries in which their hospitals are located, IHMC's medical tourist population has increased to the point that they created a medical-value travel department to work with foreign patients' home-based physicians in coordinating preventive and postoperative care, as well as assisting with travel arrangements.

Other companies have built hospitals in the geographic regions they serve. For example, Parkway Health owns fifteen hospitals across Brunei, China, India, Malaysia, and Singapore. Most of the practicing physicians are US trained, and the Joint Commission International accredits all of their hospitals. Thailand and Singapore are projected to remain prominent global medical tourism destinations due to their efficient healthcare systems with low-cost, high-quality care provided by internationally accredited medical centers with the most advanced diagnostic equipment.

The Middle East is catching up fast. Eager to gain a slice of the growing international healthcare market, the United Arab Emirates has quickly moved to bring its healthcare sector up to international standards. In addition to serving their native populations, Dubai Healthcare City (DHCC)—a zone of 120 medical facilities including hospitals, outpatient medical centers, and diagnostic laboratories—was created to attract foreign investment, offer international-standard advanced private healthcare, and become a globally recognized destination for medical care. More than 4,000 licensed professionals are employed in DHCC, and 12 million people travel to Dubai every year for healthcare services.

The amount of money at stake in the global medical tourism market is vast. Global revenues from medical tourism exceeded $56 billion in 2008. A report by Grand View Research estimates the medical tourism market will be worth $131.35 billion by 2025. The magnitude of destination healthcare can be seen in the map below, which denotes the over fifty countries with 1,060 healthcare organizations that have achieved accreditation from the Joint Commission International (JCI). These include academic medical centers, hospitals, and primary care providers.

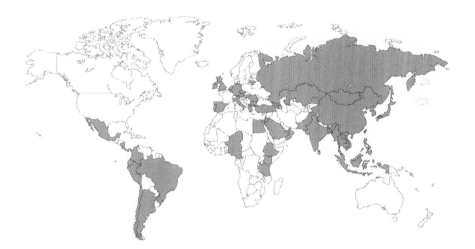

Over fifty foreign countries host 1,060 healthcare organizations that have achieved accreditation from the Joint Commission International (JCI) and provide destinations for medical treatment.

Source data for this graphic was used with permission from JCI.

The cost savings by receiving care in foreign countries is significant. The following are approximate costs (prices will vary somewhat due to exchange rate differences) and do not include travel or lodging. These are the average cost per medical procedure in the US compared to the average cost for the same procedure in thirteen countries around the world.

Medical Procedure	United States (average)	Foreign (average)
Heart Bypass	$123,000	$18,108
Angioplasty	$28,200	$8,575
Heart Valve Replacement	$170,000	$20,395
Hip Replacement	$40,364	$13,480
Knee Replacement	$35,000	$11,961
Spinal Fusion	$110,000	$13,365
Gastric Bypass	$25,000	$12,495
Hysterectomy	$15,400	$6,370

For those in the US who think India, Singapore, or the UAE are too far away, Dr. Devi Shetty (a driving force behind Narayana Health in India) has completed a 104-bed hospital on Grand Cayman Island. Known as Health City Cayman Islands, this 107,000-square-foot facility opened in February 2014, becoming that country's first advanced medical facility and tertiary care hospital. Bringing together the quality services and affordable pricing of Narayana Health with the technological innovation of Silicon Valley, expansion plans for Health City Cayman Islands include an academic institution and biotech research facility.

Health City Cayman Islands is clearly trying to grab a share of the US healthcare market by offering high-quality care on a tropical paradise less than an hour away from Gulf Coast states at a fraction of the cost of the same care in the United States. As Dr. Shetty says, "If a solution isn't affordable, it's not a solution."

DISRUPTIVE FORCE #4
THE POWER AND PROMISE OF TECHNOLOGY

Several broader disruptive technologies such as 3-D printing, artificial intelligence, blockchain, and even electric cars will impact all industries, and healthcare will be no exception. As you'll see, the only limitation with new technologies is our imagination.

3-D Printing

3-D printing is a method of manufacturing to create physical objects based on a digital blueprint. The creation of a 3-D printed object is achieved using an additive process—hence why it is also known as additive manufacturing—that involves laying down successive layers of material until the end product is created. Each of these layers can be seen as a thinly sliced horizontal cross-section of the eventual object. 3-D printing is the opposite of subtractive manufacturing, which consists of cutting out or hollowing out a piece of raw material.

3-D printing enables the creation of complex, functional shapes using less material than traditional manufacturing methods. It also enables mass customization, allowing the creation of personalized products for individual consumers, such as hearing aids. It has been successfully used to create a variety of industrial items and consumer goods such as automobiles, furniture, clothing, and even food.

With respect to healthcare, 3-D printing has been used to create instrumentation and medical equipment, implants (such as heart valves, knee and hip joints, cranial plates), medicines, external prostheses, exact models of a patient's organs, bone, and even synthetic skin.

Among the more exciting uses of this technology has been the printing of customized 3-D models of organs and body parts prior to surgery. These have enabled surgeons to look at and even practice the procedure prior to an actual operation, thereby improving the chances for a better surgical outcome. Similarly, 3-D printed patient-specific prosthetic limbs and orthotic braces are having a major impact on the lives of people, especially those who would otherwise be unable to afford them.

3-D printing is enabling high-quality, rapid, low-cost manufacture of just about everything, and innovators are currently testing its uses. According to StartUs Insights, "The healthcare industry is expected to raise investments in 3-D printing from 1.6% in 2016 to 20% by 2026. Though this technology has yet to have its breakthrough in healthcare, prosthetics and dental implants have already been printed successfully. Moreover, 3-D printing allows for the creation of personalized medication dosing as well as personalized pills. Because pills are printed in various drug layers, patients could soon be taking only one instead of multiple pills. On top of these opportunities, the most ambitious goal for this technology is the creation of living tissue and organs—a goal expected to be reached within the next 20 years."

This technology promises even more in the years to come and will facilitate, as well as enhance, the practice of precision medicine.

In practice, 3-D printing is providing twenty-first-century care. For delicate procedures, surgeons at many hospitals examine X-rays and use a generic model to discuss their plan. At Ochsner Health System (southeast Louisiana's largest nonprofit, academic, multispecialty, healthcare delivery system), 3-D printing technology enables surgical teams to print exact replicas of impacted areas so they can better prepare for the procedure.

In addition to 3-D printing, Ochsner has also been developing virtual reality and augmented reality technologies, which can create detailed soft-tissue models to help plan procedures such as heart bypass surgeries and neurosurgical procedures. These advanced medical visualization techniques also help patients understand their condition and treatment plan.

Artificial Intelligence

Technology whereby computers learn from experience, adjust to new inputs, and perform human-like tasks is called artificial intelligence (AI), machine intelligence, and cognitive computing. Most examples of AI that people are familiar with—chess-playing computers, self-driving cars—are trained to do a clearly defined task and rely heavily on what is known as deep learning and natural language processing. Using these technologies, computers can be trained to accomplish specific tasks by processing large amounts of data and recognizing patterns in the data.

The foremost limitation of AI is that it only learns from data—there is no other way in which knowledge can be incorporated. So any inaccuracies in the data will be reflected in the output.

Another limitation of AI is specialization. An AI system that can play chess cannot play Monopoly. Likewise, a system that can detect fraud cannot drive a car or provide legal advice. Even more, a system that can detect tax fraud cannot detect other types of fraud. In other words, AI systems are hyperspecialized.

Finally, AI systems are not autonomous. The fictional AI technologies seen in popular entertainment are still science fiction. However, computers that can probe complex data to learn and perfect specific tasks are becoming fairly common.

In healthcare applications, AI is not yet extensively employed, but this technology will essentially alter the way patients are treated. Within the next decade, software algorithms will disrupt current practices by carrying out tasks that generally require human intelligence. From chatbots providing diagnostics based on symptom input and automation supporting physicians in image-based diagnostics and making smart diagnoses—AI will help reduce the risk of human errors.

Artificial intelligence will never replace human beings. Like every other technology, AI will bring its strengths (to do many tasks at once, quickly perform repetitive tasks, reason deductively) to augment and complement people's natural abilities and strengths (to improvise and use flexible procedures, exercise judgment, reason inductively).

Because AI algorithms process information differently than people do, AI can see patterns and relationships that people cannot. The interaction of people with AI offers many opportunities. It can bring analytics to new domains, improve the performance of existing analytic technologies, enhance decision-making, diminish language/translation barriers, augment our existing abilities, and much more.

For healthcare, the emergence of artificial intelligence has provided unprecedented levels of data tracking and analytic capacity, which has enabled new information and insights to be readily available to consumers, providers, hospitals, insurers, and others. AI applications are already helping doctors find the right treatments for various diseases, determining the accurate dose of drugs to give to patients, providing personalized medicine and X-ray readings, helping the blind tackle everyday tasks, and even performing supervised surgery with autonomous robots.

We believe artificial intelligence will make excellent providers even better. In addition, personal healthcare assistants can act as health coaches, reminding people to take their pills, exercise, or eat healthier.

The future for AI in healthcare is as bright as it is for 3-D printing. Projects under way include efforts to predict which combinations of drugs will be most effective for specific patients, fight diseases whose treatments have not improved in decades, identify skin cancers, monitor multiple high-risk patients, and many more. AI has already delivered value to consumers and providers and will continue to do so exponentially in the coming years.

Blockchain

Blockchain is a distributed and public/open ledger that is used to record transactions between two parties efficiently in a verifiable and permanent way. Typically managed by a peer-to-peer network collectively adhering to a protocol for internode communication and validating new blocks, a blockchain is decentralized with no central administrator or centralized data storage, and records (or blocks) are linked using cryptography (techniques for secure communication). Once recorded, the data in any given record/block cannot be retroactively altered without alteration of all subsequent records/blocks, which requires a consensus of the network majority.

Although blockchain is best known for being the technology behind crypto currencies such as Bitcoin and Ethereum, it transcends financial applications and offers many solutions that are likely to disrupt various industries, including healthcare. Think of crypto currencies as the baby steps in the development of blockchain technology. By enabling bilateral financial transactions, crypto currencies are analogous to email, which enabled bilateral messaging. And just as email is a limited application relative to the broader internet technology upon which it is based, crypto currencies are a similarly limited application relative to the blockchain technology upon which they are based.

The uses of blockchain beyond crypto currencies are small but growing. The technology is already being used to bring a broader array of affordable financial services—including banking, micropayments, and remittances—to people who've never had access to them, to track items through complex supply chains, as well as for smart contracts that hold both parties accountable by only completing the terms of the agreement once both parties have fulfilled their end of the bargain.

Blockchain has the potential to become the system of record for all transactions—where all pertinent information is embedded in digital code and stored in shared, transparent databases protected from tampering, revision, or deletion.

Imagine that every patient record, every insurance claim process, every payment, every provider directory, for example, had a digital record and signature that could be identified, validated, stored, and shared. Consumers and healthcare organizations could freely and directly transact with each another, and the role of intermediaries such as accountants, bankers, brokers, lawyers, and payment processing services would be fundamentally changed—if they were even needed at all.

CB Insights evaluated emerging uses for blockchain in healthcare based on known stakeholders, projects already under way, scalability requirements, and necessary safeguards. In a recent report, they identified where blockchain will most likely be integrated into healthcare in the short, medium, and long term.

Most immediately, they believe we will see simplification of back-office operations such as managing provider information and improved traceability in the supply chain. In the medium term, we will see applications for claims management, payments, and prior authorizations; health information exchanges and research data; and research and trial design. However, some of the most exciting projects involve the wholesale reimagining of how healthcare data are accessed and owned through universal identities, patient health records and app services, although CB Insights believes these possibilities are further off.

If the aforementioned things happen, the economy will undergo a radical shift as new, blockchain-based sources of influence emerge and become part of our society's infrastructure. Blockchain must undoubtedly clear many barriers—technological, governmental, organizational, and even societal—to reach its full potential. But just as we're still finding new and creative applications for the internet after over two decades, blockchain technology is still in its infancy.

Let's take a look at blockchain in practice. Disruptor Amazon sees opportunity with blockchain technology. In November 2018, Amazon unveiled two new blockchain services: Amazon Quantum Ledger Database and Amazon Managed Blockchain.

According to Amazon, the managed blockchain offering will allow Amazon Web Services customers to set up "a scalable blockchain network with just a few clicks" that "automatically scales to meet the demands of thousands of applications running millions of transactions." Amazon's new product will support two popular existing blockchain platforms—Ethereum and Hyperledger Fabric. Ethereum is a popular open-source building platform for developers, linked to the crypto currency ether, while corporate giants including IBM are currently building projects on Hyperledger.

Electric Vehicles

Electric vehicles are propelled by one or more electric motors using energy stored in rechargeable batteries. Electric vehicle manufacturing has experienced a renaissance due to advances in batteries, concerns about increasing oil prices, the desire to reduce greenhouse gas emissions, and government incentives in the form of tax credits and subsidies.

Despite efforts to reduce the net purchase price of electric vehicles, they still cost more to initially purchase compared to vehicles powered by internal combustion engines. However, electric vehicles are less expensive to operate than comparable vehicles due to the lower cost of repairs and energy.

Electric vehicles comprise only 1 percent of automobile sales worldwide, and even less in the United States. But their sales will steadily increase as they become more affordable, as their performance, range, supporting infrastructure, and underlying technologies improve, and as a result of evolving energy needs and systems, which are becoming cleaner and increasingly decentralized—with energy generated, stored, and distributed closer to the final customers.

We mention electric vehicles as a disruptive force because of the positive health effects they will have on pollution reduction. As most people are aware, pollution from cars and trucks causes serious harm to public health. Burning gasoline and diesel fuel produces harmful gases like carbon monoxide, particulate matter, and nitrogen oxides, which contribute to serious respiratory diseases and premature death. In fact, a recent MIT study found that road transportation emissions cause 53,000 premature deaths per year nationally, making transportation the largest single contributor to premature deaths from air pollution.

Electric mobility is widely seen today as a key way to improve air quality. Electric cars driven by individual consumers, taxi operators, and used for public transportation can have a big impact in reducing pollution as well as extending and saving lives.

Self-Driving/Autonomous Vehicles

Self-driving vehicles are capable of driving and navigating without human input. Autonomous vehicles employ a variety of techniques to sense the environment, including radar, laser light, GPS, odometry (the use of data from motion sensors to estimate changes in position), and computer vision. Advanced control systems are used to interpret sensory information to identify appropriate navigation paths, pedestrians, obstacles, and relevant signage.

Although still under development, the emerging technology of autonomous vehicles is predicted to deliver a variety of benefits. From a consumer standpoint, autonomous cars will provide enhanced mobility for children, elderly, disabled, and the poor, relieve travelers from driving and navigation chores, increase traveler satisfaction, and lower fuel consumption.

From a civic standpoint, they will improve traffic flow, reduce transportation infrastructure needs, and significantly reduce needs for parking space if used in a shared manner. The potential safety and health benefits from autonomous vehicles are even more profound than for electric vehicles. These include a potentially significant reduction in traffic collisions and accidents, fewer injuries, lower costs, and less insurance needed. Autonomous vehicles will also facilitate new business models for transportation as a service, especially via the sharing economy.

Despite their vast potential, there are many challenges that will have to be resolved before self-driving vehicles become anything more than test beds. These include a host of technological issues, the safety of driverless cars, traveler and pedestrian safety, disputes concerning liability, as well as implementation of new government regulations and legal framework. Consumers will also have to overcome their psychological, emotional, and social reluctance to relinquish control of their vehicles. In addition, concerns about loss of privacy and security—such as hackers or terrorism—will have to be addressed.

Right now it is difficult for many people to envision computer-controlled vehicles roaming freely without drivers. But the day will eventually come where this disruptive potential is a reality.

Here's something to think about: "The self-driving car is coming. And right now, our best supply of organs comes from car accidents…Once we have self-driving cars, we can actually reduce the number of accidents, but the next problem then would be organ replacement," said Bre Pettis, cofounder and former CEO of MakerBot Industries (a 3-D printer company).

CHAPTER TAKEAWAYS

This chapter described some of the most compelling disruptive forces that are already reshaping healthcare, such as

» A population age wave that is hitting US shores,

» Frustrated employers who are overturning existing business models and boundaries by taking on a more proactive role with respect to the health of their workforce,

» Savvy competitors who are treating healthcare like a business, and

» Technological advancements that will improve care delivery as well as people's health.

The disruption we are beginning to experience in healthcare will render existing business models and value propositions obsolete. This will transform how people think about health and healthcare. But it also offers huge opportunities to those able to see the potential upside and who are willing to seize it. The future belongs to those who can engage consumers in creative ways, find solutions to their health needs, and deliver increasing value to them.

2

A Disruptive **Antidote**: Curing Our Ailing System in a Life or Death World

---

IN THE REVELATION OF ANY TRUTH
THERE ARE THREE STAGES. IN THE
FIRST IT IS RIDICULED,
IN THE SECOND IT IS RESISTED,
AND IN THE THIRD IT IS ACCEPTED
AS BEING SELF-EVIDENT.

—*Arthur Schopenhauer, German philosopher (1788–1860)*

It's easy to be skeptical about the notion of disruption in healthcare since we've all seen new technologies and methods appear without having much of an impact on the healthcare business. But the current wave of disruption is more fundamental, encompassing, and sweeping than anything previously seen. It is diving down to address the root causes of healthcare's woes.

There is a growing state of consumer agitation with healthcare, a groundswell of employers who are taking a more activist role in the health and healthcare of their employees, and many disruptive innovators who see opportunity and are doing something about it. These forces are poised to drive a revolution in healthcare delivery system changes.

We must unleash the power of disruptive innovation and free-market forces to shift everyone's focus from sick care to healthcare.

Nearly everyone recognizes that prevailing business models in healthcare must profoundly change. A wide range of industries—retail, transportation, manufacturing, entertainment and media, grocery—have already been deeply affected. No industry or organization, including healthcare, can afford to ignore the threat. Yet most healthcare organizations are not moving fast enough to meet this challenge. A few leaders are still in denial, others are reluctant to upend the status quo, while some simply do not know how to proceed.

This is where our book will help. So far we've described some of the most compelling disruptive forces that are already reshaping healthcare. These include a population age wave, frustrated employers who are demanding more from healthcare, savvy medical providers who are responding to employer demands by treating healthcare like a business, and technological advancements that will improve care delivery as well as people's health.

Now that we know what is happening as well as what is potentially coming, it's time for action. Here we describe what healthcare leaders can (and should) do right now to disrupt their organizations for the sake of long-term relevance and survival.

When reading the following recommendations, envision an ideal future state for healthcare. Put yourself in the shoes of consumers (which shouldn't be too difficult since we're all consumers). Accept that the ideal future for consumers and patients can become a reality, and that healthcare can be easier and less complex. Concede that consumers deserve to be empowered and have a major source of friction removed from their lives.

Healthcare leaders must acknowledge that they can choose to disrupt themselves, or wait for somebody else to do it to them.

As challenging and painful as the former will be, the latter will be even more traumatic. The trials that lie ahead will be difficult for the healthcare industry but are not insurmountable. Creating the ideal future state for healthcare will require imagination and insight as well as an obsessive focus on consumers and patients.

RECOMMENDED DISRUPTIVE INNOVATION #1
SHARE PRICES SO CONSUMERS CAN COMPARISON SHOP...LIKE WE DO FOR EVERYTHING ELSE

Would you buy a product or service—be it a pair of shoes, book, clothes, television, washing machine, mattress, automobile, or anything else—if the vendor couldn't tell you the price until after you had purchased it? Or perhaps not even until one to two months after you made the purchase? How would you feel if you found out a neighbor had purchased the same item from the same vendor but paid 50 percent less than you did? Or that people who purchased the same item from a different vendor paid 70 percent less than you did? Would you share your experience with others? Would you trust that vendor? Would you ever purchase from that vendor again?

"There is more price transparency and quality transparency regarding a refrigerator than there is about your heart surgery," said John Toussaint, MD, CEO of the Thedacare Center for Healthcare Value.

Most businesses understand their true costs and profitability, and price their products/services accordingly. They understand their cost of doing business down to the minute detail—their raw materials and supplies cost, labor costs, the cost of operating their facilities, and so on. They also understand what price the market is willing to bear for their products and services as well as what it costs to acquire and retain a customer. With this information they can make real-time, ongoing decisions about product/service mix, pricing, and marketing to ensure a steady (or increasing) flow of consumers who are willing to pay for the products and services being offered.

But healthcare is another world.

It is insane, absurd, bewildering, staggering, perplexing, and irrational. These are just a few of the terms that have been used to describe (accurately, in our opinion) the current state of costs and pricing in healthcare. For consumers, it's Alice in Medicine Land. So let's go down the rabbit hole.

The craziness begins within hospitals and providers' offices, most of which don't know what anything costs. A few might be able to tell you the cost for a specific item (Ever try getting details for an EOB (your insurance company's explanation of benefits)?). But the hospital or provider office that actually knows the bundled cost for them to produce and/or deliver a service or to perform a procedure—the accurate cost for supplies, equipment, medicine, facilities, labor, waste—is more rare than astatine (the rarest natural element on earth).

Here's a firsthand example of crazy pricing. When Terry was first hired as chief quality officer of a large hospital in the Midwest, he and the new financially savvy CEO asked the OB department to tell them how much having a baby with a normal birth (no complications, no C-section) would cost the hospital. They gave the department clear parameters, like three prenatal visits, the birthing costs, and three follow-up pediatric visits. No one had a clue. They found this to be the same in multiple departments for multiple procedures.

Often, when employers or individuals asked the hospital, "How much will that cost?" they provided a number that had been guesstimated and hoped would cover the hospital's costs. Yes, that is crazy if you are serious about running a business.

It's just as bad for the pricing of healthcare services and procedures. Medical providers have a perplexing array of prices for any given service/procedure, which are seemingly not tethered to any form of reality or logical principles. Prices are set in ways that seem arbitrary, and sometimes predatory, with little oversight and no market incentive to reduce them.

Is it any wonder why healthcare is so tortuous? Nobody anywhere in the system can tell you what something as simple as a blood test is going to cost. Not the hospital, not the doctor, not the lab doing the test, and not even the insurance company. The only supplier who could provide a price quote would be an internet company offering the same test, using the same lab, and without any involvement from the doctor or insurance company.

With respect to big-ticket items in healthcare, consumers are back in the 1960s and '70s going from dealership to dealership trying to get the best deal on a Chevy Impala. Obviously, someone in the throes of a medical emergency doesn't have time to price shop. But for consumers who can, many don't even bother to check. Some don't have time. Some rely on referrals or simply don't know where to find information. Others simply go to the hospital where their doctor practices and that also accepts their insurance.

Many don't realize a procedure can cost two to three times more at different hospitals, are unaware of how much is really being spent, and have little incentive to know the underlying costs. Further, consumers making the attempt would find it extremely difficult and time-consuming to get any healthcare provider to commit to a firm price. And consumers who do take advantage of price comparisons available through the various websites will find the preposterously expansive price ranges surrealistic.

An example of detached-from-reality medical pricing was recently publicized by NPR, who reported about a Texas teacher who recently received a $109,000 bill for care he received as a result of a heart attack. A neighbor rushed this man to the nearest ER, which happened to be an out-of-network hospital. The hospital—to whom insurance had paid nearly $56,000 for his four-day hospitalization and the procedures to clear his blocked artery—had the audacity to send him a $109,000 bill to make up the balance of their cost. After NPR made this a nationwide story, the hospital ultimately reduced their balance to $332.29, which the man paid.

Anecdotes like this leave most people dumbstruck. We're not sure which aspect of this tale is the most bizarre—the $165,000 total cost for four days of care (in comparison, four nights at a Ritz-Carlton in New York City would cost just over $4,000), or the 99.7 percent discount this man eventually received. One can only surmise the best way to secure an almost 100 percent discount for an outlandish medical bill is to go public and shame the medical provider.

Stories about insane medical pricing abound (for example, $25,000 for a thirty-minute MRI, $17,850 for a urine test, $14,018 for stitches on a finger, $5,751 for an icepack, $629 for a Band-Aid) and illustrate just how far away from a true economic market the healthcare system has become. They reveal the unreality that healthcare now is.

Does anyone think $165,000 for a four-day heart attack–related stay is reasonable? What is the actual cost for the hospital to provide this service? Does the price vary depending on which insurance a patient has? Should consumers routinely experience bewilderment and frustration when attempting to find pricing for healthcare, or apprehension at the arrival of a bill?

Numerous factors contribute to the current, untenably high healthcare costs, where consumers' pockets are picked by the healthcare industry without them even realizing it. Some of these are outside the control of healthcare leaders. Because most Americans receive health insurance through their employers, and because employees do not pay taxes on employer-paid insurance premiums, the tax system has created an insidious cost hiding mechanism that subsidizes employees receiving health insurance through their employers, placing them at an advantage over others who must purchase health insurance on their own.

Further, because employers often pay a significant portion of the total health insurance bill, many employees behave as if their health costs are borne by their employers and have little incentive to shop around and compare prices. It's only when they start receiving surprise bills that they are galvanized to action, albeit too late. Another factor is the lack of transparency regarding what insurance companies pay hospitals and providers for their services.

...the healthcare industry has made it difficult for patients to act as healthcare consumers.

In other words, the healthcare industry has made it difficult for patients to act as healthcare consumers.

So let's consider whether people can really be consumers of healthcare. Naysayers would argue that it is unlikely people will ever become consumers of healthcare, even if prices were transparent and people had the means to compare them. Certainly, no one would be shopping around from the inside of an ambulance. However, according to a 2017 Hoover Institution report by Scott Atlas, emergency care represents only 6 percent of health expenditures. For privately insured adults under sixty-five, almost 60 percent of spending is on elective outpatient care, for which informed choice and proper incentives would reduce costs.

Likewise, nearly 60 percent of Medicaid money is spent on outpatient care. Atlas even notes that for the top 1 percent of spenders—a group responsible for more than a quarter of all health expenditures—a full 45 percent of spending is on outpatient care. Giving people an incentive to consider price and value when seeking such care would turn them into consumers and go a long way to reducing costs.

There are undoubtedly other factors, but these are broader issues we will not dive into here. Our concern is what healthcare leaders are in a position, and have the power, to do right now.

What can healthcare leaders do to prevent consumers from having any more Alice in Medicine Land experiences with respect to pricing? What can healthcare leaders do so consumers are not forced to act in ignorance of, and against, their own economic interests? What can healthcare leaders do to begin to rectify the inexcusably high costs of healthcare?

Consider the characteristics of healthcare's ideal future state for consumers regarding costs and pricing. This is what we described in the imagine section at the beginning of the book:

> » Consumers can easily access the information necessary to make informed choices about health and healthcare for themselves as well as for family members/loved ones.

> » Decisions are based on meaningful comparative data, not on a physician's or hospital's general reputation, the experiences of friends, or where a physician has admitting privileges.

> » Consumers are empowered and able to seek out the most cost-effective care with the best outcomes without worrying about being in or out of network.

> » Consumers know exactly what each physician and hospital across the country charges for standard procedures and what their bill will be when they make a choice.

With this in mind, there are three things healthcare leaders can (and should) do now: know the real costs, reduce pricing variability, and reduce the opacity of prices.

Know the Real Costs

One of the most fundamental tenets of developing and growing a business is to know how much it costs to produce a product or deliver a service. It is fundamental because such information allows companies to price their products and services, ascertain the profitability of each, prepare budgets, and identify opportunities to control their costs.

"There is no method to this madness," according to William McGowan, former CFO of the University of California–Davis Health System in Sacramento. "As we went through the years, we went through these cockamamie formulas. We multiplied our costs to set our charges."

Melanie Evans chronicled the efforts of one hospital to better understand its costs for knee replacement surgery in an investigative article in the *Wall Street Journal*. Like many other hospitals, this one routinely raised the price for this procedure by an average of 3 percent a year. In 2016, the average list price was more than $50,000, including the surgeon and anesthesiologist.

According to Evans, an eighteen-month review was performed where an efficiency expert trailed doctors and nurses to record every minute of activity and note instruments, resources, and medicines used. They also tallied the cost of nursing time, mismatches of available post-surgery beds, unnecessary and costly bone cement, as well as delays dispatching physical therapists to get patients moving. Their actual cost, including physicians, turned out to be $10,550—five times lower than the list price.

What the aforementioned hospital did was akin to cost accounting, which is a tool to help leaders understand the costs of running a business and make decisions. As an internal reporting system, the costs associated with producing products and/or delivering services are classified, tracked, and recorded based on functions, activities, products, and process. Cost accounting is analysis-based and may combine objective and subjective assessment of the costs contributing to a standard output. Although ubiquitous in most industries, cost accounting is more uncommon in healthcare.

This knee replacement story is one example of where a hospital was ignorant of its actual costs, and exemplifies the need for all healthcare organizations to know every expense they incur to deliver the services and perform the procedures they do.

The day is coming (sooner than many think) where employers and consumers will demand to know bundled prices for every product, service, and procedure.

For medical providers who do not already have a cost accounting system in place, this should become one of their highest priorities. We have witnessed and experienced the implementation of cost accounting systems in healthcare. Although the process is laborious and time-consuming (especially for the finance and accounting staff), the information available from such systems is more than worth it.

Many people have shared their experiences with insane healthcare pricing on Reddit, a social news aggregation, web content rating, and discussion website. We can't vouch for the accuracy of everything on Reddit, but the palpable disdain for healthcare pricing is a frequent topic. If you've never been on this site, we encourage you to take a look just to see what people are saying. Some of it will make you angry, and some of it will make you laugh.

Reduce Pricing Variability

Many have seen studies and data illustrating extreme variation in the cost of care across the country. Astronomical price ranges for many common procedures have become widely publicized in healthcare. For example:

Treatment of breathing problems
(less than four days in hospital)
from $78,000–$273,000

Heart failure
from $7,304–$173,250

Total hip replacement
from $11,100–$105,000

Pneumonia (simple case)
from $5,093–$124,051

Appendectomy
from $1,529–$186,955

Knee replacement
from $24,000–$47,000

Endoscopy
from $600–$7,700

The problem is equally pervasive within the same metropolitan areas, where hospitals' prices differ by staggering degrees for the same procedures just a few miles away:

Lower joint replacement | Dallas
from $42,632–$160,832

Lower joint replacement | Washington, DC
from $30,000–$69,000

COPD | New York City
from $7,044–$99,690

Knee replacement | Miami
from $27,115–$44,237

Lower back MRI | San Francisco
from $475–$6,221

Pregnancy ultrasound | Cleveland
from $183–$522

Even within hospitals, charges for the same procedure can vary wildly based on whatever deal the hospital has made with different insurance companies.

If that's not maddening enough, looking across countries routinely shows significant disparities between what American consumers pay compared to the average cost consumers bear in other countries. Here are just a few examples for procedures of varying complexity as well as common diagnostic tests:

Heart bypass surgery
US = $78,318 vs. Spain = $14,579

C-section
US = $15,240 vs. Netherlands = $5,492

Appendectomy
US = $13,910 vs. Australia = $5,177

Normal vaginal delivery
US = $10,808 vs. South Africa = $1,271

Colonoscopy
US = $3,059 vs. Australia = $372

MRI
US = $1,119 vs. Spain = $130

CT scan of the abdomen
US = $1,301 vs. Spain = $85

In case you're wondering, US consumers pay much more on average—often double—for all health services, procedures, diagnostic tests, and medicines than consumers in other countries. The incredible variation in pricing is a signal that competitive forces are out of whack in healthcare, which in turn is driving the explosion of overall spending on the industry. The current levels of spending as well as the upward trajectory must, and ultimately will, be reversed.

Healthcare prices vary for a variety of reasons, including differing overhead costs, variation in provider practice patterns, market dynamics, and, in some instances, a need to offset the costs of complex services by billing higher rates for simpler ones.

We're not saying every hospital should charge the exact same amount for a given procedure or service. There are competitive differentiators (such as better clinical outcomes, lower morbidity, a more established program, better technology, a better residency program, etc.) that warrant a premium. But we are saying that the old cliché "you get what you pay for" simply doesn't exist in healthcare, and that more expensive care is not always better care.

There is little justification for one hospital to be charging two, three, four, or more times what another is for the exact same procedure with the same clinical outcomes. There is absolutely no justification for the same hospital to be charging two, three, four, or more times for the exact same procedure based on someone's insurance. The price is not right when it comes to medical costs in America. In fact, it's nowhere near right.

Reduce the Opacity of Prices

The way reimbursement is negotiated among insurers, hospitals, doctors, and other providers—along with the pricing for most healthcare services and procedures—is largely hidden from employers and consumers. And because very few in the industry know what anything actually costs, pricing is divorced from the reality that a competitive market would bring.

As consumers become more responsible for paying the fees for healthcare services, they will need (and they deserve to have) reliable, clear, and accessible pricing in advance. As employer-sponsored health plans continue to evolve, consumers will increasingly insist upon price transparency. Besides, how many patients are hospitals losing to retail clinics, stand-alone surgical centers, and providers delivering direct primary care? To remain competitive, the visibility of pricing and other information consumers require for assessing value must be radically improved. It must become much more transparent, accessible, and defensible.

Dave Brat, US Representative from Virginia, said this: "If you take your kid in for the sniffles, you pay $20, but the full cost is $200. And so we need to get back to the price system where you see the full cost of healthcare, and then people will make smarter decisions. That will reduce healthcare costs, and it's a huge part of our economy."

As of January 1, 2019, hospitals and long-term care facilities were required to post their charge masters online. Known as the inpatient prospective payment system (IPPS) and long-term care hospital prospective payment system (LTCH PPS), these are attempts by the Centers for Medicare & Medicaid Services (CMS) to create patient-centered healthcare by providing greater price transparency so patients have what they need to be active healthcare consumers.

Increased price transparency is certainly a step in the right direction, but this rule will cause problems for consumers in the short run because the prices contained in hospital charge masters are hyperinflated and bear no resemblance to the prices ultimately paid for care. In addition to actual costs of services, procedures, and overhead (none of which most hospitals really know to begin with), charge master pricing routinely includes some guessing regarding profit, unpaid collectibles from patients who were uninsured and could not pay, operating losses across the hospital, inefficiency in how the hospital was being operated, and a host of other unrelated expenses.

The reality is that the shamefully inflated prices on charge masters are intended to be a starting point for hospitals to enter negotiations with health insurers. If an insurer demands a 50 percent discount, hospitals can say yes knowing it will still be making money because they threw everything including the bathroom sink into the charge master price.

We urge providers to go beyond the 2019 CMS rule. Providers need to figure out what their actual cost is, add a profit margin that sufficiently accounts for the quality of care and service differential provided, make that their standard price for anyone and everyone regardless of their insurance or employer, and make the pricing widely available in consumer-friendly ways.

Do it and keep it simple. Do it to empower patients with cost and quality information. Do it to create the type of value-based system and more transparent pricing that Amazon, Boeing, Cisco, Comcast, Disney, Walmart, and the like are already providing to their customers, are looking for from healthcare, and that other large employers (and eventually consumers) will soon be demanding. Do it to lead the industry.

Though this type of pricing is challenging to implement, some healthcare providers are beginning to provide standardized pricing for a number of common services and procedures. INTEGRIS Health System (Oklahoma City, OK) developed a tool that provides price estimates for common outpatient procedures. Not only does the tool provide accurate quotes, but it also helped improve patient communication and, when appropriate, steer patients to lower-cost providers that operate within its network.

Advocate Health Care (Downers Grove, IL) instituted a "Jiffy Lube" model of posting standard prices with add-on charges for extra services. It also posted flat prices for an array of services for self-pay patients at its urgent care clinics and outpatient centers. And St. Claire Hospital (Pittsburgh, PA) posted a pricing tool on its website to help consumers estimate out-of-pocket costs based on their insurance plans.

In addition, many insurers offer comprehensive price-comparison tools so consumers can compare their individual out-of-pocket costs for procedures at different hospitals.

The most famous of all heart surgeons, Denton Cooley, MD, offered this thought: "Of the many 'firsts' with which I have been involved at the Texas Heart Institute—including the first successful human heart transplant in the United States and the first total artificial heart transplant in the world—the achievement that may have the greatest impact on healthcare did not occur in the operating room or in the research laboratory. It happened on a piece of paper…when we created the first-ever packaged pricing plan for cardiovascular surgical procedures."

> **30 percent of medical bills are incorrect and the kindest thing we can say about them is that they are baffling.**

Since we're talking about price transparency, let us also mention billing. As things currently stand, 30 percent of medical bills are incorrect and the kindest thing we can say about them is that they are baffling. For many, trying to understand an explanation of benefits (EOB) is Dante's fourth level of hell. Is it possible to make them 100 percent correct? Is it possible to simplify these mystifying and irritating things?

We think so, and as part of our crusade for clarity, we ask hospitals to consider the ideal future state for consumers regarding billing where billing for health-related care is straightforward, and bills are clear, easily understood, and known in advance. We all demand nothing less for every other product and service we purchase, so why not for our medical services as well?

Ryan Grassley became nationally known (and will long be associated with insane hospital billing) after he used Reddit to post a photo of an itemized hospital bill he and his wife received for the birth of their child. Their bill contained a $39.35 charge for "skin to skin after C-sec." The post attracted more than 12,000 comments along with national media attention. The visceral loathing for the hospital charging a young couple to hold their own newborn baby was widespread. People commenting wondered how much the hospital charged the couple to name their baby or to take him home. The Grassleys later disclosed the name of the hospital and said they were more amused than outraged by the charge.

Get Doctors Involved

Everyone agrees that making healthcare more affordable is a good idea. But what few people realize is that physicians (unlike other medical providers) ultimately determine how 90 percent of healthcare dollars are spent. Given the consumerization of healthcare, patients will increasingly expect providers to look out for their wallets the same way they expect providers to look out for their health.

It is challenging for clinicians to know how their decisions will impact what patients pay. In addition, having clinicians take responsibility for protecting patients' wallets requires new skills, training, and tools. Fortunately a nonprofit called Costs of Care is dedicated to helping prepare medical providers to look out for patients' healthcare-related finances by considering unintentional financial harm from the medical decisions providers make as they address patients' clinical needs.

Costs of Care is helping to transform American healthcare delivery by empowering patients and their caregivers to deflate medical bills. High-value medical decisions benefit individual patients and society at large, and Costs of Care sees an opportunity to return $100 billion to the American people by trimming the fat out of medical bills. They seek to accomplish this by helping medical providers replace or reject services that eat into consumers' wallets without making us healthier.

Just as the patient safety movement helped clinicians think about how to prevent unintended physical and emotional harm, a new movement is under way to help clinicians think about preventing unintended financial harm.

Considering all the aforementioned recommendations, we believe it is possible for the effectiveness of healthcare to be improved to the point where the United States has more than enough money to treat every American needing care.

RECOMMENDED DISRUPTIVE INNOVATION #2
PROVIDE EASY ACCESS TO CARE WHERE AND WHEN CONSUMERS WANT IT

Ensuring consumer access is an important component of the patient care tapestry and is a critical element of the healthcare value proposition. Access is the starting point for all consumer encounters with the healthcare industry. If a person cannot access care, not only is it impossible to receive medical attention, but it's also impossible to build relationships with medical care providers and achieve overall wellness. Unfortunately, consumer access to care is not a reality for many people across the country.

As we see it, to make healthcare less expensive, more accessible, and easier to use, care will have to be moved to the most appropriate skill level, including the patient, and to the most appropriate site, including the home.

Offering sufficient and convenient access to healthcare services presents numerous challenges for providers, including limited appointment availability and office hours, geographic location, transportation issues, consumer awareness of their care options, and clinician shortages. Any of these can negatively impact consumers' health and well-being.

Health providers who offer appointments during traditional work hours (Monday through Friday from 8:00 a.m. to 5:00 p.m.) or have only limited afternoon and evening availability may be inaccessible for the majority of people who work during these times as well as for parents with children who attend school. Consumers need office hours that allow them to see healthcare providers outside their normal work or school schedules.

Geographic location is another challenge. Consumers living in rural areas are the most likely to face challenges in accessing adequate healthcare because they are more likely to have to travel long distances to access healthcare services, especially for specialist services, than people living in an urban or suburban area. This can pose significant burdens in terms of time and money and often causes people to go without adequate care. In addition, those living in rural areas are typically more confined due to lack of available treatment facilities.

The lack of reliable transportation is another barrier to care that can impact the health and well-being of consumers. Transportation is a basic and essential step for ongoing healthcare and medication access, especially for people with chronic diseases that require regular provider visits, medication access, and ongoing changes to treatment plans to ensure good care and outcomes.

> ... accessing care is not about getting a foot in the door, but about getting a foot in the *right* **door.**

In addition, transportation is increasingly being recognized as a key social determinant of health. Those living in rural as well as urban areas who do not have access to reliable transportation are more likely to delay or forgo healthcare altogether, miss appointments, and abandon proper medication use. These factors in turn increase health-related costs and lead to poorer health.

Consumers also need to be aware of the various care options available to them. Often, accessing care is not about getting a foot in the door, but about getting a foot in the *right* door. It is important for healthcare organizations to make sure consumers understand how to get to the proper care setting, and we're not referring to travel directions.

Healthcare providers are increasingly integrating alternative treatment sites into their service mix, such as urgent care centers, retail clinics, and freestanding emergency departments. But while more care options are a positive step for accessing care, it is important for healthcare providers to educate patients on the appropriate settings for common medical needs.

Finally, it's a given that without people to provide care, patients can't receive it. Shortfalls of nurses, doctors, and other clinical staff have always been a challenge within the healthcare system, but are becoming an increasing concern. The aging population, staff retirements, and insufficient numbers of new medical care providers being trained are a few of the factors causing what appears to be a permanent labor shortage in healthcare for both clinical and nonclinical staff. Staffing shortages create stress and burnout among staff as well as lead to inconsistent care and mistakes that make providing high-quality, affordable care an overwhelming task. This is a big challenge that healthcare is trying to rectify.

The aforementioned barriers will be a formidable challenge, but should not prevent consumers from seeking appropriate care. First and foremost, healthcare organizations should keep in mind what consumers want. In an increasingly consumer-centric healthcare system, it will be important for healthcare organizations to offer access to care in ways that are convenient for consumers.

Next we share a number of patient-centered mechanisms that healthcare organizations are employing to ensure consumers can easily access the appropriate care services. These are novel, out-of-the-box approaches some healthcare organizations are already taking to make things easier for consumers.

As you read them, consider what the ideal future state might look like for consumers. The imagine section of the book outlined that ideal picture:

» Consumers can access care (in a simple and stress-free way) when and where it is most convenient for them, including through digital channels like email, apps, social media, and other eHealth platforms using video conferencing/telemedicine.

» Consumers will not have to wait a week for an appointment, experience long waits to see a provider, or nervously wonder which of the people sitting around them in the waiting room is the most infectious.

» Consumers receive routine physicals and checkups using technology in their homes with equipment that monitors vital signs in real time and provides alerts to them and their designated provider if anything needs attention.

» If face-to-face consultation is required, provider visits to consumers' homes will supplant visits to the office, clinic, or emergency room as the default option.

» If an office or clinic visit is necessary, a wide selection of choices is available nearby via neighborhood clinics in nontraditional locations (such as retailers, grocers, and workplaces) as well as at provider offices with no appointment necessary and little, if any, wait.

Provide Patient Transportation

Transportation plays an essential role in the quality of life for consumers in the US. It is a critical component in obtaining adequate food and clothing, education, employment, as well as for social activities. With respect to healthcare, barriers to transportation have a big impact on people's health as well as the quality of care they receive.

We're all familiar with the problems caused by patients who lack adequate transportation, including missed or late appointments, going off medication regimens, and even discharge delays from inpatient settings. Fortunately, there are emerging ways to counteract this issue that healthcare organizations have begun to employ.

Ride-hailing companies Uber and Lyft (featured among the disruptive organizations highlighted earlier) are helping to close care gaps arising from medical transportation issues. Uber has started its own healthcare offshoot (aptly called Uber Health), and Lyft has partnered with Allscripts to help patients connect with rides to medical appointments. Healthcare organizations have also been forging their own relationships with Uber, Lyft, or other niche medical transportation services.

One of our clients—Denver Health Medical Center—wanted to reduce the no-show rate for outpatient visits as well as the time patients waited post-discharge to travel to their next destination (whether that was home or rehab). After conferring with patients, they confirmed lack of transportation was a major reason for these problems.

Denver Health explored and then abandoned the possibility of adding a new multistory parking garage (at a cost of nearly $26,000 per space), before offering free bus tickets, cab vouchers, and a private car service using a donated vehicle staffed by volunteers. Denver Health subsequently started collaborating with Lyft to provide vulnerable patients transportation to and from the hospital. Initially limited to patients in the emergency department, it was later expanded to hospital inpatients.

The initiative now includes outpatient clinics and is expanding based on the community's needs and suggestions for improving practices. Denver Health uses Lyft for hundreds of patient rides each quarter and has moved the needle toward their goal of reducing missed appointments and wait times for patients leaving the hospital and its clinics.

Providing transportation for patients is an excellent example of the type of community health partnerships that help keep patients healthier. And since it works for patients, how about for staff? We guarantee subsidized Uber, Lyft, or similar service for staff will be less expensive than a parking garage at $26,000 per space.

Use Augmentation Clinics

Let's face it, schlepping to some far off medical office is a hassle. You'll probably spend more time finding a parking spot than with the medical provider. How much more convenient would it be to go to a nearby retailer or grocer for medical care? Somewhere you could walk to from wherever you live. Somewhere you could just show up without an appointment. Somewhere you wouldn't have to wait too long to see a provider. Somewhere the staff weren't stressed out.

If medical providers haven't already partnered with a nearby retailer or grocer to launch an urgent care clinic to augment their emergency department (ED) and other outpatient centers, they should consider doing so. This will provide relief to their ED/outpatient center staff, ease the strain on their facilities, and provide a convenient outlet in which nonemergency patients can receive easy-to-access, fast, and affordable care.

Southeastern Regional Medical Center (Lumberton, NC) has done so with very good results. Recognizing that many people who show up at the ED are not emergency cases, they partnered with a local Walmart to open an urgent care center inside the retailer to handle nonemergency care.

The clinic only has one exam room, and service prices are clearly posted—a physical is $25, and for patients without insurance, a sick visit is $65. Patients can also get their prescriptions filled immediately at Walmart's pharmacy. The clinic is staffed by nurse practitioners and handles noncomplex ailments like sinus infections, colds, and the flu.

The staff are capable of performing more complex procedures such as suturing and abscess drainage, but only if there is no one else waiting. Patients who need more advanced care can be sent to one of the hospital's larger, more full-service clinics where staff can provide X-rays, set fractures, and perform other services not available at their Walmart clinic. The clinic has helped ease the stress of long wait times (the average time from arrival to leaving the clinic is under fifteen minutes) and costly care.

As Andrew J. Sussman, MD, president of MinuteClinic and senior vice president/associate CMO for CVS Caremark, said, "More than 50 percent [of our MinuteClinic patients] are effectively medically homeless. Patients at MinuteClinic did as well or better than those treated in traditional primary care settings, yet cost was 40 to 80 percent lower than in other settings."

Use Telemedicine/Telehealth to Enable Virtual Treatment

Healthcare organizations are also overcoming access barriers by using communications technologies to enable patients to seek medical advice without needing to come into traditional medical settings (such as the office, clinic, or hospital). Telemedicine allows patients to refill prescriptions and receive medical treatment, medical monitoring, coaching, and training remotely from any distance, without needing to physically be present. This benefits patients by allowing them to seek care closer to home, remain near family during care, lose less work time, and reduce travel costs.

Telehealth technologies include telephonic communication, videoconferencing, internet conferencing, email, and streaming media. So long as a patient has a phone or computer with internet connection, they can use telemedicine services.

Telemedicine is especially helpful in expanding access to care for people who live far away from a clinic or hospital as well as those with busy schedules who may not otherwise be able to see a doctor during normal office hours. Full-time workers can use telemedicine to conduct appointments during the workday. Parents can access providers via telemedicine, helping to ease burdens that can arise when a child becomes sick. Imagine not having to pack up all the kids and schlep to a doctor's office for an appointment. Likewise, the elderly can connect with medical providers without having to leave their homes or nursing homes.

Healthcare providers can also use telemedicine to connect with specialized experts as needed. This helps patients avoid the hassle of traveling great distances to receive intensive or specialized care using tools only available at larger organizations. Telemedicine can also be set up to provide text messages or emails aimed at educating consumers, providing medication alerts and reminders, and schedule a check-up and provide information about available resources. Such text messages can be automated or initiated by a health provider.

An exciting aspect of telemedicine is the use of remote health monitoring devices that feed information to medical providers about their patients' heart rates, blood pressure, and other vital signs. If the provider sees a spike in blood pressure, for example, they can send a text message or call the patient to engage that person and recommend a course of action. The intersection of wireless technology, health-related apps, and healthcare providers has opened new degrees of accessibility and will continue to expand (one example is Apple's new watches have a heart monitoring feature).

With growing cost pressures and significant unmet medical needs, the use of telemedicine can extend the reach of physicians and other care providers, enable clinicians to work at the top of their license, and make it easier for patients to access the healthcare system. Offering convenient, easy-to-access care options—and keeping patients out of waiting rooms—will also translate to a better patient experience and increased patient accountability.

> ...the use of **telemedicine** can extend the reach of physicians and other care providers...

Here's how telemedicine works in real life and, in this case, serves an entire state. In 1999, Mississippi had few trauma centers and ninety-nine acute-care hospitals, three-quarters of which were in rural areas with no more than twenty-five beds and located more than thirty-five miles from another facility.

The acute-care hospitals had no specialists on staff, performed no surgeries, and even lacked labor and delivery units because they had no obstetricians. Many lacked imaging equipment required to diagnose emergent conditions, and none had a ventilator. Patients requiring serious emergency care were often transported from those hospitals to the University of Mississippi Medical Center (UMMC) in Jackson, an expensive and medically risky solution.

As a result, the trauma center in Jackson was always overcrowded. There was an endless stream of patients who had traveled some distance seeking care, sometimes at great risk. Kristi Henderson, UMMC's clinical director of nursing in the ED, asked a couple of insightful questions, "Why not reverse the flow? Why not build capacity in the rural clinics by sharing the medical expertise concentrated at UMMC through a telehealth system?"

Just as Henry Ford used the assembly line (which was a significant manufacturing disruption of that day) to make automobiles less expensive and more accessible, UMMC used telehealth to accomplish the same with respect to the healthcare for the citizens of Mississippi.

Henderson was realistic about how impossible it would be to secure a state-funded, top-down telehealth effort. So being a savvy realist, she began a pilot project to link the trauma team in Jackson with the primary care doctors and nurse practitioners who staffed most of the critical access hospitals. The local practitioners would process admissions, stabilize patients, perform simple procedures, order lab work and EKGs, and take basic images. The emergency team in Jackson would observe the patients on dedicated TV screens, read the X-rays and other images, diagnose the problems, talk the local practitioners through the treatment plans, and be available for follow-up care, either in person in Jackson or remotely through the network.

Once fully developed, this TelEmergency network concentrated the scarcest expertise and equipment in the Jackson hub, which handled advanced procedures, while the community hospitals would serve as gateways and service points (in other words, as the spokes) for simpler procedures. The telehealth network saved money by reducing patient transfers and treated more people in local hospitals where costs were as low as half those at UMMC. The network also helped keep small, financially insecure hospitals afloat by increasing their emergency room services and revenue streams.

What Kristi Henderson began in three pilot community hospitals in 2003 has expanded significantly. Today the UMMC telehealth network provides thirty-five specialty services to more than 200 hospitals and service centers, including schools and prisons, throughout Mississippi. Because of this pioneering disruptive work, an entire state and many thousands of lives were positively affected.

Although UMMC helped pioneer telehealth in the early 2000s, similar efforts are under way in other states. As just one example, the University of Nebraska Medical Center in Omaha is using telehealth to reach eighty rural nursing homes to make available one (of five in the state) geriatric psychiatrist who can diagnose and treat nursing home patients as well as coach staff in those facilities to deal with behavioral issues without medicine.

In addition, Children's Hospital and Medical Center of Omaha reaches kids across Nebraska using telehealth to provide access to a pediatric psychiatrist who can connect with the children and their parents in their primary care provider's office. By going to their primary care doctor in a small, rural town—and linking up electronically to the specialist who is hundreds of miles away in Omaha, in a separate room with a computer screen—no one is the wiser why the child is seeing the doctor, thus reducing the stigma surrounding mental health.

There's also a mobile app for parents to use for quick medicine checks with the psychiatrist at Children's Hospital. These are typically short Facetime-type encounters parents can use during the course of their busy days. Kids simply leave school and meet Mom in the parking lot, hop in the car, Facetime with the psychiatrist, and head back into school in fifteen minutes.

Use Digital/Virtual Assistants to Help Consumers Foster Healthy Behaviors

The increasing use of personal digital assistants like Amazon's Alexa, Apple's Siri, Microsoft's Cortana, and Google Assistant illustrate how far commercial applications of language and speech technology have progressed in recent years. These digital assistants are popular across all age groups and are used in voice-driven products like Amazon Echo and Google Home as well as our smartphones. Many consumers leap at the prospect of having a personal assistant perform mundane tasks like finding information, checking the weather, ordering food, making reservations, and many others just by saying a few well-chosen (and carefully pronounced) words.

In the context of health and healthcare, personal assistants have the potential to enable a much higher level of connectivity and interaction among consumers and providers. Healthcare has numerous opportunities to provide a launching pad for these technologies to be used for improved patient outcomes.

First and foremost, digital assistants can be used to assist patients with their care. For patients who are being monitored outside the hospital due to a recent discharge or as part of ongoing care for a chronic condition, it can be cumbersome to continuously track their condition through mobile devices and applications. A digital assistant will offer these patients more flexibility by capturing data through their voices. By using natural language processing optimized for healthcare, virtual assistants will better understand patients' needs and conditions and will have more meaningful data to report back to healthcare providers.

That help can come in the form of digital assistants. Digital assistants are already being used to provide reminders for routine tasks like taking medications, checking blood pressure, checking blood sugar, or putting on a life alert pendant. They can also be used to schedule doctor appointments, monitor various signs of a person's own health (such as number of steps taken each day or heart rate), research various health-related topics, request information, place a call to a care provider, summon emergency medical care, and even to conduct drop-in visits with family members and loved ones who agree to give each other access. This enables people who need to check up on someone not living with them to use their digital assistants as a built-in intercom system.

> ...personal assistants have the potential to enable a much higher level of **connectivity** and interaction among consumers and providers.

The refinement and expansion of personal digital assistants will continue with more innovations. What began with mobile devices and desktops will soon move to televisions and other electronic devices with which we interact. People may soon have a virtual butler who knows their likes and dislikes, or a virtual doctor who knows a person's health circumstances and attempts to improve their quality of life—and perhaps nag about the extra serving of cake. The goal of healthcare virtual assistants is to empower people to live healthy and independently with peace of mind that assistance is nearby.

The use of digital assistants within virtual reality (VR) environments is another intriguing concept to think about. VR is an interactive computer-generated experience that takes place within a simulated environment. It incorporates mainly auditory and visual feedback, but may also allow users to grasp items. This immersive environment can mimic the real world with astonishing fidelity and is already being used in clinics to treat addiction, anxiety, depression, and other disorders.

One company, BehaVR, is using VR to create experiences that activate cognitive, emotional, and physiological responses with the goal of improving health. BehaVR experiences empower individuals and lower barriers to health with personalized educational content, emotional regulation skills, and stress reduction techniques. The BehaVR program has delivered improved emotional and physiological responses in patients.

We have both experienced VR and were impressed not only by its realism and capabilities but also its potential healthcare applications. In one instance, Terry visited a calming beach environment that was beyond relaxing. Virtual therapists came into the scene from time to time to make suggestions about how to relax or go deeper into a state of meditation. The company sponsoring the demonstration said that virtual physician visits with real doctors would soon be possible.

VR is beginning to make significant improvements to the lives of people with autism, chronic pain (reducing the need for medication), traumatic brain injury, memory loss, anxiety, phobias, and even psychosis. Furthermore, medical care providers can help relax hospitalized patients, enhance care, and reduce boredom of the elderly.

The possibilities of VR in healthcare seem endless, and much experimentation is taking place. For example, an interesting use of VR is in the restoration of low vision (which affects 135 million people globally). Low vision cannot be corrected by surgery, medicine, or glasses, and severely affects the patient's ability to do their everyday tasks. Up until now patients had no other choice but to just live with it. Products like IrisVision help low-vision patients regain their sight via VR experience.

We Are Alfred is a VR-powered product created by Embodied Labs that aims to let young medical students understand what it is like to live as a seventy-four-year-old man with visual and hearing impairments.

VR is also being used to enable medical students to explore the inside of virtual bodies to see each organ as it relates to the overall bodily system. VR can bring the learning and teaching experience in medicine to a higher level by allowing surgeons to stream operations globally. Medical students, on the other hand, can use VR to step into the operating room and see every procedure down to the last detail.

Use Mobile Clinics to Bring Healthcare to Consumers

There's been a spotlight on the mobile health revolution that makes it possible for consumers to see their doctors from their kitchen or office. But there's another mobile health application that doesn't fit in the palm of your hand or on a desktop. It's much larger and looks like a cross between an RV, a rock star's bus, and a doctor's office. It's a mobile health clinic, and it affords healthcare providers a nimbler platform to connect with the communities they serve.

Many healthcare providers and private companies around the country are taking mobile health literally. They're customizing RVs, vans, buses, and ambulances with telemedicine tools and wireless connectivity. Some mobile units boast multiple exam rooms, a dentist's chair, and capabilities for doing lab work. Functioning like a satellite clinic, people climb in, check in, and are seen by medical providers just like a normal clinic.

Mobile clinics will enable medical providers to offer basic services closer to where they are needed. This includes schools, businesses, and underserved communities. Mobile clinics will reduce time to treatment, help push population health initiatives, and make life easier for consumers.

Mobile clinics have been around for decades, but they are experiencing a renaissance as they assume a more prominent role in delivering preventive care that is affordable and more easily accessible. Mobile clinics also allow hospitals to shift their focus to managing chronic illness and preventive care to keep nonemergency cases out of their ER. By traveling into the community and offering affordable services, mobile clinics remove logistical constraints around transportation, making appointments, wait times, and administrative processes.

Mobile clinics also overcome more subtle barriers in maintaining good relationships between medical providers and community members by fostering trusting relationships that allow staff to stay engaged with community members and to support them through behavior changes as well as to help them navigate the healthcare system.

Mobile clinics have a critical role to play in providing high-quality, low-cost care. They represent an integral part of the healthcare system. Mobile clinics improve access, bolster prevention, and enhance chronic disease management.

Thinking smaller and even more convenient, mobile devices (mHealth) are a key component of the eHealth revolution and signify a drastic shift in consumer behavior. In 2017, 1.7 billion people downloaded health-related apps, illustrating the increasing demand for such tools. Services such as remote monitoring, evisits, and eprescribing are all enabled by mobile devices and applications. Though mHealth offers advantages such as improved outcomes and reduced costs, securing devices and apps will be a challenge. Start-ups working on security technologies will help to improve confidence, which is key to successfully implementing mHealth solutions.

Access to medical services is ultimately about meeting patients' overall needs. By making themselves conveniently available to patients, medical providers can ensure that patients receive treatment regardless of their circumstances. As the industry becomes increasingly consumer-centric, medical providers will need to adopt more flexible approaches, ensuring plentiful access to healthcare services.

Take Healthcare into Patients' Homes

Traditional healthcare settings (such as acute-care hospitals and outpatient clinics) will always have a place in medical practice since they are essential for handling medical conditions requiring specialized, highly technical, and intensive care. But these settings are not always the best for chronic or nonintensive conditions.

A major drawback to hospitals is that they are germ factories. With the rise of antibiotic-resistant bacteria, every patient entering a hospital runs the risk of contracting an infection. Indeed, at any time, one in twenty-five patients is battling a hospital-acquired infection.

Providing care to patients in their residences is another way to deliver convenient medical treatments without the risks associated with hospitals and without the up-front costs of mobile health clinics. House calls are not a new concept—they date back to the 1930s, when visits to patient homes were prevalent. In fact, it was not uncommon for a doctor to go into a patient's home if they were too sick or injured to seek outside medical attention. Not only was this opportune for patients (no travel, no waiting), but was also less costly while enhancing patient health and well-being.

In today's era of disruption, it may be easy to dismiss such a quaint practice. But modern communication technologies and portable medical tools are causing a renaissance of this old-fashioned way of providing service.

Many consumers are under the mistaken impression that home health is only available for individuals who are homebound. Some physicians may not even realize which patients are eligible for and would benefit from such care. Although home care is ideal for those who are confined to their homes, the reality is that receiving care at home can benefit people in many other situations, including those who are experiencing changes in how they're able to complete daily activities, adjusting to a new diagnosis or new medication, undertaking rehabilitation after surgery, or suffering from dementia, Alzheimer's disease, or age-related cognitive changes. Of course, home care can simply be offered as a convenience for any patient.

Nurse practitioners, physician assistants, or physicians, if necessary, can deliver home care. Other members of the care team—nurses, physical therapists, speech therapists, and occupational therapists—can also deliver specialized care. The types of services that can be provided at home (or at the office) are many and include physicals and wellness visits, lab work, chronic care management, wound care, and others.

> **[home care] provides a clear and unique perspective of the patient's surroundings and health issues...**

Beyond consumer convenience, one of the most significant benefits of home care is that it provides a clear and unique perspective of the patient's surroundings and health issues, thus giving the medical care providers a more holistic perspective with which to provide a careful diagnosis and proper treatment options for the whole person.

It's also being shown that home care can be delivered at lower cost and with better outcomes. Studies show that hospital-level care at home for certain conditions can be provided for 30 percent to 50 percent less than inpatient care with fewer complications, lower mortality rates, and higher patient satisfaction. In addition, because it is provided in comfortable and familiar surroundings, home health may encourage more people to see a doctor.

Here's something interesting to consider. Prospective car buyers no longer have to go to a dealership to test drive a car. Using the Hyundai Drive app, prospective car buyers can schedule an at-home test drive for any of the automaker's vehicles. The car will be brought to your home (or office or favorite coffee shop or wherever you prefer), and you can take a test drive with a company representative. If Hyundai can do it, so can healthcare.

Technology solutions are being developed that will complement and facilitate home-based care. These will make home care a practical reality for many consumers. For example, cardiologists at BJC Healthcare and the Washington University School of Medicine (WUSM) in St. Louis know that heart failure (HF) patients are at risk for developing excessive fluid retention, which results in shortness of breath, fatigue, and other medical problems. Often, these patients require hospitalization to reduce their fluid levels. Such hospitalizations could potentially be avoided if signs of fluid retention could be detected early enough to initiate home-based treatments.

Dr. Thomas Maddox, a cardiologist himself and executive director of BJC/WUSM's Healthcare Innovation Lab, says prior efforts to detect early signs of fluid retention have been largely unsuccessful due, in part, to the excessive burden it places on patients to provide a substantial amount of information about symptoms, weight, and other health information to their care team.

In an attempt to improve this process, the Lab is working with an outside company on home-based HF monitoring, which involves a bed-based sensor that requires minimal input from the patient. The sensor can detect heart rate, sleeping patterns, and other early symptoms by passively monitoring patients while they are in bed. These data are then analyzed using machine learning techniques to determine which signals can detect early HF problems. If fluid retention or other problems appear to be developing, the patient's care team can be notified, and treatments can be instituted. This project will test the accuracy of the sensors and design clinical care pathways to manage the information.

Ultimately, this sort of monitoring program could extend the reach of the care team, improve patient satisfaction, and reduce adverse clinical outcomes for HF patients as well as those suffering from other conditions.

Here's another example. Medically Home Group is a technology-enabled acute-care substitution service focused on the 25 percent to 30 percent of patients currently in hospitals who could be cared for at home. Through clinical collaborations with nonprofits Atrius Health and VNA Care, and by integrating evidence-based pathways and various in-home devices, Medically Home ensures patients receive the highest levels of care surrounded by their family at home, or as the company calls it, "micro-hospital unit in the home."

The Medically Home model provides an asset-light, care delivery model that uses both the resources and infrastructure of the hospital and the patient's home to substitute for the currently disconnected and costly inpatient hospital care, post-acute care (such as skilled nursing facilities), and readmission/episode prevention (population health) services.

Medically Home's technology is HIPAA compliant and can be integrated with electronic medical records for live monitoring and clinical data processing. Medically Home aligns the imperatives of financial, clinical, and service delivery transformation to achieve health system sustainability, and their model promises a reduction in the total cost of care, better clinical outcomes, reduced readmissions, and a significant enhancement to existing population health programs.

RECOMMENDED DISRUPTIVE INNOVATION #3
OUR BODIES BELONG TO US, NOT YOU: LET PROVIDERS BE HEALTH PARTNERS

Becoming and being a medical provider of any type—doctor, nurse, therapist, or one of the many other care-oriented occupations—takes time, dedication, and hard work. But these vocations can be tremendously fulfilling and invigorating.

There are as many reasons people go into healthcare as there are people going into the field. Most go into healthcare with a genuine altruistic desire to help others. They want to have relationships with people and yearn for the opportunity to care for them and to help them stay healthy. They want to blend science, psychology, and artistry to make a difference in people's lives. They want to fight diseases. And they feel a duty to guide people toward healthy, happy lives. These are some of the brightest and most talented people in the country, and we are fortunate they are called to healthcare.

Unfortunately, those idealistic hopes and dreams quickly and vividly collide with the administrative, procedural, and economic aspects of today's healthcare system.

Every day, scores of mundane administrative chores disconnect medical care providers from the reasons they chose healthcare as a profession in the first place. There are too many rules and regulations to be aware of and followed, never-ending documentation requirements, countless forms to check off or complete, note writing and coding visits, documenting informed consent and warding off liability, chart audits, time-consuming attempts to obtain prior authorization for a procedure, and other skirmishes with insurance companies.

For many providers, it seems they spend more time performing these nonmedical tasks than they do interacting with patients. Combined with the uncertainty that is more prevalent in today's healthcare industry as well as more acute patients, it is becoming more difficult to practice medicine, and the environment is overwhelming. It's no wonder burnout is a frequently discussed topic among health professionals.

There is no doubt that working in healthcare is both thrilling and frustrating. So what can everyone do to help medical care staff get back to spending the majority of their time focusing on things that add value to consumers, to help healthcare providers have more meaningful interactions with people, to reduce the need for fast-turn appointments, and to reduce the gatekeeper role primary care physicians often play?

Bear in mind our look at the ideal future in the imagine section of this book:

» Providers think of themselves as—and act like—consumers' health coaches, counselors, and advocates.

» Providers acknowledge that people's bodies belong to them, not the providers.

» Providers partner with and include patients (and their families when appropriate) to ensure that that healthiness and well-being are part of everyone's daily routines, to prevent illness, and to jointly discuss and resolve any health issues that arise.

» Providers use the most current, scientifically sound information and technology to help diagnose and treat their patients, using an evidence-based approach rather than eminence-based.

» Providers know as much about nutrition and other healthy interventions as they do about prescribing medications.

» Since no one can learn everything they need to know in medical school, providers have trouble-free access to artificial intelligence and digital assistants to augment their knowledge and to help with diagnosis and treatment.

» Providers are aware of and consider consumers' socioeconomic situations and basic resource needs when making prevention and treatment recommendations.

» Providers feel energy and excitement every day as they spend more time with patients and less time performing administrative tasks.

» Providers have also abandoned white coats, so they do not make people feel inferior or delude themselves that they are somehow superior.

Fine-Tune the Supply of Health Providers and Move Tasks to the Most Appropriate Skill Level Including the Patient and Family

Fundamentally, without staff to provide healthcare services, consumers can't receive them. In our current system, a number of barriers inhibit the efficient and effective delivery of care to patients, and in some cases artificially worsen shortages of staff. Staffing shortages create stress and burnout among healthcare providers as well as lead to inconsistent care and mistakes that make providing high-quality, affordable healthcare services an overwhelming task. This is a big challenge that needs to be rectified. But what should be done?

The supply of medical providers should be significantly yet strategically increased. With enough medical providers operating at the right levels of training, consumers will have options to evaluate so they can choose the best value for their money. Having overqualified medical staff delivering services is wasteful, inefficient, and contributes to both the shortfalls of doctors, nurses, and other clinical staff as well as to increased costs.

Our experience is that physicians are overtrained to perform 50 to 60 percent of the procedures they do, including many primary care tasks (such as routine physicals, administering vaccinations, and dispensing common drugs). A study by the Hoover Institution found that 88 percent of clinic visits involved only simple care. These services can and should be performed by medical care providers with a more appropriate skill level, such as physician assistants or nurse practitioners. Not only would this ameliorate some of the staff shortages, it would significantly reduce healthcare costs and enable physicians to focus on patients with more acute needs.

In addition, a report from the Medical Group Management Association showed that nonphysician providers are extremely effective at driving patient satisfaction as well as easing patient volume off physicians.

For years studies have proclaimed physician shortages in the United States. A 2018 report by the American Association of Medical Colleges predicted a shortage of between 42,600 and 121,300 physicians by 2030. They further indicate shortages will occur in both primary and specialty care, and that specialty shortages will be particularly large. The main evidence cited for the shortage is that the supply of new doctors isn't keeping up with changing demographics—chiefly a growing and aging population—along with the retirements of older physicians.

There is no doubt that the United States does not have enough physicians; however, the situation need not be as desperate as some portray. While supply is not keeping up with population growth, alleviating the physician shortage will require a multifaceted approach. One is shifting care to the most appropriate level. Another is the introduction of team-based care, where physicians work with nurses, dentists, pharmacists, social workers, and even public health professionals to address the needs of their community and ensure patients receive the right care.

Better use of technology (such as telehealth and remote monitoring) to make care more effective and efficient, increasing use of nonphysicians, and reducing the number of unnecessary treatments and procedures will also help ease the shortfall. Some healthcare facilities in India use videos to train family members to take care of the patient while in the hospital so they can learn the skills under supervision and continue it once the patient gets home.

Providing care for less cost is possible in the right setting with the right staff. A friend of ours took a position as CEO of a hospital where the previous administration had planned an addition to the hospital that would have cost $1 billion. After careful study of this plan and current trends, including the outmigration of care from the hospital to the clinic, the new CEO knew that the future was in moving work to the appropriate skill level and to the appropriate setting. So he revised the plan and built a state-of-the-art ambulatory care center for $250 million, saving the hospital and community $750 million while providing the care that was actually needed.

Obviously, it pays to understand the forces driving new, disruptive ways of thinking and not just do what has been done in the past, which is often driven by outdated underlying belief systems.

Hire Health Coaches and Make Them a Priority

The challenges to medical care providers posed by people with chronic conditions are immense. Another desperately needed change that will improve the health of the population as a whole and reduce the burden on providers is the use of health/life coaches to work with people as intensively as necessary to help change their unhealthy behaviors.

For decades, countless studies have shown how a few preventable behaviors—poor diet, physical inactivity, tobacco use, and alcohol consumption—place people at an increased risk for type 2 diabetes, cardiovascular diseases (such as heart attack, high blood pressure, high cholesterol), stroke, chronic obstructive pulmonary disease (COPD), some cancers, and premature death. In fact, more than 70 percent of deaths in the US result from chronic conditions, and approximately 75 percent of healthcare dollars are spent fighting chronic diseases.

Further, indirect costs such as absence from work, low productivity, disability, and poor quality of life add to the personal and economic burden of chronic illnesses and are significant contributors to increasing demands on the healthcare system. Not only have these unhealthy behaviors developed into the leading cause of disease, they have become the dominant health issue of our time.

The strong causal relationship of lifestyle choices and unhealthy behaviors on illnesses and chronic diseases is crystal clear. And most people understand the link between lifestyle choices and their own health. However, far too many people choose unhealthy behaviors anyway. They overeat. They are sedentary. They smoke. It's not uncommon to hear "It tastes so yummy" or "It makes me feel good" or "I can't change," with little regard for the overall effects of that attitude on themselves, family members, friends, the larger community, and the healthcare system.

Even Thomas Edison pictured the future a century ago when he said, "The doctor of the future will no longer treat the human frame with drugs, but rather will cure and prevent disease with nutrition."

Fortunately, people do have help. Medical providers and public health agencies provide plenty of information on the impact of lifestyle choices as risk factors for preventable diseases and encourage individual responsibility for health. In addition, many communities, businesses, and schools have jumped in to make environmental and systemic changes—including walking trails, bike lanes, exercise programs, smoking cessation programs, more healthy meal options, and others—to encourage and reinforce healthy behaviors. The objective is to help people replace unhealthy habits with healthy ones in order to maintain wellness and prevent illness and disease.

Unfortunately, these efforts are not enough. Seeing and understanding the link between lifestyle choices and health is easy enough, but changing our own long-established, traditional behaviors is significantly more challenging. Just ask anyone who has ever made a New Year's resolution, or who struggles to maintain a healthy lifestyle while balancing work and family.

We must be honest and acknowledge that (1) people's unhealthy behaviors lead to significant health problems, (2) behaviorally caused health problems account for a significant portion of our country's total healthcare expenditures, and (3) most people need extensive help to change their behaviors.

People do not act without reason. Every action we do or do not take, and every choice we do or do not make, is related to conscious or subconscious needs. Becoming aware of these motivators is difficult for many people, and using that information to affect change is beyond most people's capabilities. This is where health/lifestyle coaches can and should play a role. Coaches can work one-on-one or with groups to help people understand the drivers behind their unhealthy choices and to transition them to a healthy lifestyle through mindful, internally driven behavior changes.

> **Every action** we do or do not take, and every choice we do or do not make, is related to conscious or subconscious needs.

The good news is coaching works, and people can experience significant as well as sustainable health improvements by making small changes to their daily activities and taking responsibility for their own health.

Wellness coaches are at the forefront of an influential shift in helping people improve their health as well as their lives. Health coaching has moved beyond simply counseling people about nutrition or teaching proper exercise techniques. It has become focused on behavioral change and helping people establish the right mindset. Most people already know what to do to be healthier; the problem is they aren't doing it.

Health coaches have evolved into masters of behavior change. Healthy habits create healthy results, and the most effective health coaches do not prescribe a one-size-fits-all approach or tell clients what they should or should not do. Instead, they help people create lifestyle changes that are sustainable and effective for them. The goal is for people to make naturally better choices for themselves so they can be happier and more balanced in all aspects of their lives.

Practice Evidence-Based Medicine

We frequently hear medical professionals speak of evidence-based medicine. In fact, we see a persistent and widespread belief among medical staff that all patient care is delivered based on the most current, best available scientific evidence, and that the efficacy of whatever treatments are being delivered has been proven. Unfortunately, for all the remarkable benefits contemporary medicine offers, the evidence suggests that evidence-based care is often not delivered. In fact, an astonishing number of treatments that research has shown are ineffective or even dangerous are routinely delivered to patients.

Sometimes providers haven't kept up with the research. Other times they know the scientific findings but continue to deliver these treatments because they seem intuitive, they're popular and widely known, they're more afraid of doing too little than of doing too much, as a defensive move in the event of a lawsuit, and even because patients demand them. In other instances, medical care providers succumb to the availability heuristic—the human instinct to base important decisions on an easily recalled, dramatic example.

Medical providers, like all people, vividly remember the heartbreaking case—the scan, the test, the operation that they *should* have done—because it sticks with them. Hence even consummate professionals with the best intentions tend toward overdoing things. When contradicted by evidence, these medical practices remain the standard of care, often for many years.

The literature is replete with studies, books, and articles about the lack of evidence-based practice, and the numbers are staggering. Researchers in Australia identified 156 current medical practices that were most likely unsafe or ineffective. Another analysis published in *Mayo Clinic Proceedings* reviewed ten years of original articles published in the *New England Journal of Medicine* and found that approximately 40 percent of current medical practices (146 out of 365 examined) may be ineffective and should be reconsidered.

A few examples of ineffective medical practices found by the authors include:

» Stenting for stable coronary artery disease—a multibillion-dollar-a-year industry—was found to be no better than medical management for most patients with stable coronary artery disease.

» Hormone therapy for postmenopausal women that was intended to improve cardiovascular outcomes was found to be worse than no intervention.

» The routine use of the pulmonary artery catheter in patients in shock was found to be inferior to less invasive management strategies.

The result is that many people in the United States (and around the world) have been subjected to overtesting and overtreatment in one form or another, incurring huge costs in the process while putting themselves at risk. The fact of the matter is that much of what the healthcare industry is doing simply doesn't help patients. The unintended consequences of inappropriate care include both physical and financial impacts. Millions of people are taking medications that aren't helping them, undergoing procedures that will not make them better, and receiving scans and tests that not only have no benefit for them, but also often cause harm.

Unnecessary care artificially crowds the system by tying up providers who are less available to see the patients who truly need help. And the financial impact of unnecessary care robs every household of thousands of dollars each year, consuming money that would otherwise be spent on life's necessities (such as shelter, food, clothing, and education), invested, or saved.

Striking the proper balance between innovation and effective care is incredibly difficult. Once practices are in place, they tend to persist even in the face of contradictory proof. Like many industries, medicine is quick to adopt practices based on inconclusive or preliminary evidence because they are shiny and new, but slow to drop them once they've been disproven by empirical evidence. However, the repercussions are more serious when providing medical advice to consumers and care to patients.

Medical caregivers should undertake regular, careful reviews of the research that has been published in their areas of practice. They should review information provided by organizations such as the RightCare Alliance and the Cochrane Collaboration that are attempting to bring medicine back into balance—where everybody gets the treatment they need, and nobody gets treatments they do not. They should consult with their colleagues at least quarterly to review the findings and determine where and how practice changes should be implemented. And at the very least, providers should cease performing the numerous medical practices that have already been thoroughly debunked.

About twenty-five years ago, for example, there was much pressure to reduce C-section rates and increase vaginal births after C-section (VBAC) rates. We saw some progress then, but have witnessed a significant rebound over the years. We were targeting about 20 percent back then. The World Health Organization now says 10 percent to 15 percent is a good target. Another recent study in the *Journal of the American Medical Association* says 19 percent is more appropriate. The US is currently running at 32 percent, so either way we're far above any recommended level.

To highlight the problem, we share the experience of our colleague's son. He happens to be an ED physician and his wife is a nurse. For each of their three children they were adamant that C-section was the absolute last resort to be used only if Mom or baby were in true danger. Yet the pressure on them was great to schedule a convenient delivery and resort to C-section on a hair trigger. These were highly trained healthcare professionals who had clearly expressed their wishes to their medical team, yet they had to fight to not have C-sections for each of their children.

Provide Digital/Virtual Assistants to Providers

Medical providers, especially physicians, are spending more time performing administrative functions associated with patient care and less time interacting with patients. Dissatisfaction and burnout are common topics among providers, and many wouldn't recommend the field to young people considering pursuing medicine as a profession.

We haven't met a single medical provider who wasn't yearning to spend more time with patients. All would cheerfully give up the keyboard and mouse to do more of what they went into medicine for in the first place. Likewise, we've yet to meet a patient who wanted less face time or a less positive interaction with their provider.

Fortunately, a number of commercially available AI-powered digital technologies have become available to reduce the administrative burden on providers. They are voice-activated virtual assistants—think Apple's Siri or Amazon's Alexa, but for healthcare providers—specifically designed to increase provider efficiencies and improve patient experience. These virtual medical assistants can help book appointments; retrieve patient information, test results, and imaging files; chart physician notes; place orders; and even create action plans for patient care based on the physician-patient visit and the physician's known preferences and clinical practice guidelines.

Virtual assistants can also help with billing, claims management, and inventory. When linked with the EHR, all of these things can be accomplished through voice recognition technology without touching a keyboard or mouse.

Imagine being able to predict critical medical events before they happen. That is the goal of the newest artificial intelligence tools developed by the innovationOchsner (iO) team. Combining complex machine learning algorithms and Ochsner's Epic electronic health record platform with the computing power of Microsoft Azure cloud, Ochsner has created a powerful tool that can predict patient deterioration and alert a rapid response team who can proactively intervene to prevent adverse events. Such events might include sepsis, wrong-site surgery, treatment-related infections, falls, or even mistaken identity.

Ochsner is one of the first health systems in the country to use this type of technology to improve patient care, and early results have been exceptional. During a ninety-day pilot period, cardiac arrests and other adverse events outside of the ICU were reduced by 44 percent. As Ochsner continues optimizing this technology, the system expects to be able to detect health patterns, learn from its insights, and develop more aggressive preventive measures and proactive treatment plans, ultimately preventing many adverse events before they happen.

The real benefit of digital assistants is that they can accompany physicians throughout a patient visit, augment and complement their knowledge, and ensure mistakes are not made. If the physician thinks of something, they can document it immediately. If the physician is creating progress notes and a care plan, the virtual assistant can extract the orders from the plan, create orders on its own, and confirm the orders with the clinician. Further, virtual assistants can make suggestions and ask questions during the patient encounter, when appropriate. Such artificial intelligence assists the physician and helps to ensure an error-free encounter with every patient.

For anyone concerned about negative effects of digital assistants on providers, the American Medical Association's executive VP and CEO, James Madara, MD, expressed it well when he said, "The future is not about eliminating physicians; it's about leveraging physicians. Leveraging [physicians] by providing digital and other tools that work like they do in virtually all other industries—making our environments more supportive, providing the data we actually need in an organized, efficient way, and saving time so we can spend more of it with our patients."

Artificial intelligence technology has advanced far and can handle the important, yet time-consuming clinical documentation and medical orders, freeing up clinicians to shift their focus back to patients. And as we all know, clinicians who spend more time with patients are seen as being more concerned and invested in their patients and tend to receive higher patient satisfaction scores.

Virtual assistants have significant potential in improving clinical processes and outcomes. It is a young technology, and further research is required to assess their value and ensure full benefits from their widespread use. They must fit into the regulatory landscape, and the accuracy of voice recognition is a major challenge. But when these are solved, digital assistants will unshackle healthcare providers from electronic health records and bring them back to the joy of medicine: interacting with patients.

Medical professionals have long had to keep up with a continuous flow of treatment innovations and new clinical information. Dr. Toby Cosgrove, former CEO of the Cleveland Clinic, stated in a news interview, "The total amount of knowledge in healthcare is doubling every 73 days; 5,600 journals put out 800,000 articles a year. No doctor can keep up with that. There is more information in one mammogram than there is in the New York City phone book. There are increasing amounts of information coming from genomics and elsewhere. Companies are coming together and saying that once information is in the cloud, they will share it. Going to the cloud facilitates interoperability, which enhances the ability to apply machine learning and Artificial Intelligence. This could help outcomes, increase quality, and reduce costs."

> "The total amount of knowledge in healthcare is **doubling** every 73 days..."

Further, he said, "MIT is focused on AI and machine learning and is devoting $1 billion to building a whole new campus just for the study and teaching of AI."

We believe AI will greatly enhance the ability of providers to diagnose and provide excellent care, but not replace them. Others may disagree. Time will tell.

Move to a Primary Care Membership Model

What do Netflix, Pandora, Dollar Shave Club, Stitch Fix, Zipcar, Costco, and Amazon (of course!) have in common? If you're not familiar with any of these highly successful businesses, just ask a teenager or young adult. Each of these companies is based on a membership model or offers premium memberships where consumers pay a subscription to gain unlimited access to products or services.

Far from its humble origins at country clubs and gyms, the membership-based business model is expanding at a rapid pace in many industries and is dramatically transforming the way consumers purchase a variety of products and services such as movies, music, razors, clothing, on-demand access cars, and many other goods.

Netflix and Costco are two of the most well-known examples of how member-based businesses are transforming consumer-purchasing habits and disrupting traditional practices. And these businesses are thriving amid much upheaval because they not only provide superior products and services, but also in large part due to their membership fees.

In case you aren't familiar with Costco, members pay $60 a year for a basic membership or $120 for an executive-level membership (that includes extra savings and increased cash-back benefits from purchases) for access to the retailer's approximately 760 warehouses around the world. Almost 75 percent of Costco's operating profits come from those yearly fees. Further, the retailer's renewal rate is 90 percent, proving that most customers are happy to pay for the privilege of shopping at the retailer and enjoying its wide selection, generous discounts, and weekly food samplings.

All the companies using a membership-based model try to unleash the power of data on purchasing history for the benefit of consumers, but few do it more effectively than Netflix and Pandora. These organizations use real-time analytics to track purchases and build a profile of a consumer's likes and dislikes. As the algorithms get to know a consumer based on their purchases, they produce recommendations that fit a person's particular tastes and personalize the experience for them. As anyone who watches programs on Netflix knows, the more you watch, the more pertinent the recommendations become.

Cost savings are the primary reasons for consumers to subscribe to a product or service or to purchase a retail membership. But why would a business want to pursue a membership-based approach? Here are a few reasons why membership models can benefit almost any organization:

» Memberships generate stable, predictable recurring revenues, which in turn create financial stability and certainty.

» Memberships provoke perceived value. By paying an annual fee, consumers feel like they're savvy shoppers. Why not spend $50 now to save $300 during the year?

» Memberships create the perception of exclusivity. By delivering superior products and services and/or by creating memorable experiences that aren't available elsewhere, members have access to new features or benefits that most other people aren't entitled to. This makes members feel special.

» Memberships foster brand loyalty. After paying a membership fee, consumers have a strong reason to concentrate their purchasing where they are members.

» Memberships nurture ongoing relationships and regular visits. Memberships represent an ongoing and potentially long-term relationship, which not only boosts loyalty but also increases the sales of other goods and services.

» Memberships build a strong customer base. Multiply memberships by the thousands or tens of thousands and you have a cadre of brand-loyal consumers who not only keep coming back but also spread the word to family, friends, and professional acquaintances.

» Finally, members or subscribers generate data and valuable insights. Given the ongoing and often long-term nature of memberships, the data generated by members can be used to provide organizations with both reliable and valuable insights into consumer behaviors and preferences. Whether it is understanding preferred appointment times and days, or discovering busy or slow periods, the consistent data members generate enables organizations to make informed, data-driven decisions.

Let's look at that concept in practice in healthcare. On January 10, 2019, Louisiana officials announced their intent to move toward a subscription model to pay for expensive hepatitis C treatments. Instead of paying for each prescription individually, the state is seeking to pay a subscription fee to a drug manufacturing partner to obtain unlimited access to the drug. The goal is to help end the state's hepatitis C epidemic—affecting over 39,000 people in the state's Medicaid program and in its prisons—that kills more people than all other infectious diseases combined.

In 2018 the state spent $35 million to treat 1,000 people. When successful, Louisiana's effort will demonstrate the power of membership/subscription models to dramatically decrease costs for care and treatment.

In March 2017, *Business Insider* reported on a movement happening with primary care doctors called direct primary care. Instead of accepting insurance for routine visits and drugs, direct primary care doctors charge a monthly membership fee that covers what the average patient needs, including visits and drugs at much lower prices. This is certainly a different twist on doctor-patient relationships. Consumers have to pay more up front, but also have a clear picture of how much they're spending on healthcare. Doctors can focus exclusively on their patients, simplify basic office visits, and experience significantly less stress by not having to deal with insurance companies.

An even more personalized, higher-touch approach is concierge medicine. Also called retainer-based, luxury, or boutique medicine, concierge providers typically serve wealthy individuals who place a great value on their time as well as people with complex medical conditions. In return for a higher monthly fee—which covers the cost of visits, all tests and procedures in the office, house calls, and just about anything else other than hospitalization—concierge providers limit the number of patients they see and offer enhanced access, longer appointments, and highly customized patient care. As such, concierge medicine is a more exclusive and more expensive type of membership model.

Like the membership model, concierge medicine is designed to promote doctor-patient relationships, increase face-to-face time, reduce physician workload, instill in patients a sense of personal responsibility for their health, and combat administrative waste hefted onto providers by the complexity of the healthcare system.

Membership and concierge models have the potential to eliminate the time, effort, and money spent dealing with insurance plans and billing. This in turn reduces the need for administrative and support staff. Also, since patients spend as much time as they want with their provider, they have their questions answered, which reduces the need for follow-up.

Patients within a membership/concierge model need to have insurance for catastrophic medical events. Fortunately, high-deductible health plans fit neatly into the membership-concierge business model. Although the cost for concierge care can be high, it is worth the convenience for a segment of the population. Also, the return on investment could potentially be high if consumers can forestall chronic conditions through coaching on optimal health behaviors and/or weaning off medications.

The reach of member-based businesses seems almost limitless—from razor blades (Dollar Shave Club) to music streaming (Pandora and Spotify) to entertainment (Netflix) to retail (Costco, Sam's Club, Stitch Fix) to grocery delivery (Amazon). Why not healthcare?

RECOMMENDED DISRUPTIVE INNOVATION #4
MAKE CLINICAL SETTINGS WARM AND FRIENDLY PLACES TO HEAL (AND TO WORK)

Traditional healthcare settings (such as acute-care hospitals and outpatient clinics) will always play a prominent role in medical practice since they are essential for handling medical conditions requiring specialized, highly technical, and intensive care. But the physical environments in these settings are often cold, sterile, impersonal, and intimidating. They are not conducive to enhancing health, healing, and well-being. Nor do the designs of these spaces foster the kindness and compassion of staff, or a holistic approach to meeting patients' needs of mind, body, and spirit.

In addition to their negative effects on patients, such designs often cause stress and fatigue for medical providers and staff members, undoubtedly contributing to the burnout many of them feel. For any setting in which healthcare is to be provided, new thinking is required to create a truly patient-centered environment where patients feel nurtured, where patients' education, personalized choice, dignity, and control are supported, and where staff feel engaged and empowered.

In the late 1970s an organization called Planetree was founded to help healthcare organizations create healing environments in which patient-centered care could be provided. Planetree provided a philosophy as well as an approach to care that has been adopted by nearly four hundred hospitals around the world.

Their approach is summed up like this: Person-centered care is more than hospitality. It is more than amenities and inviting surroundings. Person-centered care creates positive impressions and satisfying experiences, but beyond that, it improves lives. Person-centered care creates workplaces that energize and inspire joy at work. It improves health outcomes and unites communities around health and wellness.

Following the Planetree philosophy, everything in the clinical setting is evaluated from the perspective of the patient. Every element of the organization's culture is assessed based on its impact on patient experience, whether it enhances the humanization, personalization, and demystification of healthcare, and how information is made available to consumers, enabling them to be informed partners in their own care.

Like Planetree, think back to the opening statements about imagining the ideal healing environment:

» If nonemergent inpatient care in a hospital is necessary, patients are greeted warmly and escorted to a room upon arrival.

» The hospital itself is a place of healing beauty instead of sterile, ugly hallways and rooms.

» A physician-nurse-pharmacist triad counsels the patient, clearly explains what will most likely happen each day, orders any necessary services, and identifies an estimated discharge date.

» Any staff member who subsequently enters the patient's room identifies himself or herself, explains what they will be doing and why it is needed, performs their tasks, and asks if the patient has any questions or needs anything else.

» Patients are able to order nourishing and healthy snacks/meals a la carte whenever they are hungry.

» The physician-nurse-pharmacist triad confers with patients daily to review progress, adjust the treatment regimen as necessary, and discuss the discharge process as well as post-discharge instructions with the patient.

» Before patients leave the room, someone from the care team thanks them for entrusting their care to the hospital and its staff.

Humanize Care

Few would disagree that a supportive, caring environment for patients, families, and staff is essential to providing quality care. After all, we are human beings caring for each other, and we all have the ability to positively impact everyone we encounter. The daily interactions of medical providers with patients as well as each other should provide solace and support.

Consider a healing environment in which everyone who interacts with patients calls them by their name and introduces themselves. Patients are asked to call medical staff by their preferred name. Everyone entering a patient room introduces themselves and explains why they are there, what they will be doing, and how it will help the patient. A soft touch can also make a big difference during a hospitalization. Treating patients and visitors like guests in a home will go a long way to minimizing the intimidation factor as well as reducing their stress. In addition, hospitals should consider offering hand and foot massages (physical touch by volunteers) to help reduce stress so patients' bodies and minds have a chance to heal.

People need to be needed, and that doesn't change regardless of age or how healthy (or sick) we are. Medical providers should recognize the importance of family, friends, and social support during stressful times and should do everything possible to encourage visitation and accommodate these needs. They should also enlist family members to participate in routine care and education whenever possible to support their loved one during convalescence.

Support from volunteers should be maximized so they can play an important part in the daily routine of the hospital and enhance the services provided by clinical and nonclinical staff. Volunteers can help to make patients' stays as pleasant as possible by performing various tasks such as delivering magazines, newspapers, books, mail, get well cards, flowers, and much more.

Finally, the importance of a sense of responsibility cannot be overstated. Having plants or pets for patients to care for can also help humanize their experience. In his book *Being Mortal*, Dr. Atul Gawande recounted a story where after a doctor and staff moved several resident dogs onto their unit, patients who had been withdrawn and nonambulatory became more active and proactively (and often) began walking the dogs.

A perfect example of humanizing care is this one. On the second day after surgery, a patient was in immense pain trying to recover from the surgeon's surprise eleven-inch incision, out of which tubes were awkwardly hanging. And this pain was in spite of the medication. Prior to surgery, he had been told there would be no more than a two-inch incision, but once they got in there, they found the stone was embedded in the kidney—no longer a simple procedure.

The night after surgery, at 2:00 a.m., the patient awakened and realized he was drenched in sweat from the morphine. The air conditioner was blowing cold air across his body. His groggy thinking was about potential pneumonia and how he didn't need that, so he pushed the intercom button to summon a nurse. There was no answer for five minutes so he pushed the button again. Another ten minutes passed and still no answer, air still blowing directly on him, and chills increasing.

Too exhausted to get angry, but beginning to feel a little desperate, he hit the button a third time. A voice, in an irritated tone, came through the intercom. "Yeah, what do you want?" And the nurse took thirty minutes after that to finally get to the room.

To add insult to injury, the next morning, a healthcare assistant came into his room and set down a container of warm water on his tray. She tossed a wash rag at him and said, "Here, wash yourself," to a patient that needed ten minutes to plan a move from one side of the bed to the other to avoid excruciating pain. It is hard to imagine such pain if you have not experienced it.

As a result, this normally rational, well-adjusted patient was beginning to experience helplessness and the attending depression. He tried to tell the physician about his lack of care, but the physician was in a hurry and was more interested in telling than listening. He was a busy, important man.

Finally, on the third day when the patient was completely exhausted from little rest and even less healthcare, an angel walked into the room. She was an aide, a healthcare assistant with twenty-three years of experience of caring, yes, caring for and about people.

She said, with a beautiful smile, "Oh, honey, let me help you." She rolled up a pillow and gently tucked it in the right spot to give the patient the support he had needed for three days. Then she took a washcloth and carefully bathed him and straightened up his room, bringing the needed order that the others carelessly ignored. While she did this, she talked to him and asked about what he was experiencing. She asked about his family and joked with him, making him laugh, which hurt. But it was a good hurt. She was so authentic, so real. This beautiful sixty-year-old woman cared, really cared, and for the first time, according to this patient, the healing began.

Create Healing Environments

Medical providers should strive to create environments that are warm and welcoming with design focused on patient comfort and removing barriers between patients and staff. The experience at hospitals following Planetree design principles has demonstrated that taking a holistic view of a facility's physical space, including the total sensory environment of sight, sound, touch, and smell, can have a positive impact on patients' health, mood, and safety; aid in the prevention of disease; and provide a restorative benefit for busy medical staff members.

Using natural light, plants, art, music, and scents (or removing problem odors) is a powerful yet subtle way to create a warm and uplifting environment for patients and staff. Creating a pleasing and positive care environment that is physically and spiritually satisfying is enormously beneficial for patient and staff well-being, and surroundings that reduce stress and engage the senses are highly therapeutic for patients.

An increasing body of research is finding relationships between the physical environment of a care setting and patient and staff outcomes. In a project funded by the Robert Wood Johnson Foundation, researchers from Georgia Tech and Texas A&M analyzed thousands of scientific articles and identified more than 700 studies that establish how hospital design can positively affect clinical outcomes. A variety of factors were analyzed, including the type of lighting, ventilation, noise levels, and use of ergonomic furniture.

The researchers found strong evidence linking patient-friendly hospital designs with improved patient safety, reduced patient stress, reduced staff stress and fatigue, and overall improved healthcare quality. That our physical environment affects our emotional and physical well-being seems like common sense. Who among us is not more relaxed in a pleasant environment, or moved by the sight and smell of beautiful plants and flowers, or by a captivating painting?

Personalize Care

Taking a holistic view of patient care, personalized healthcare is much more than precision medicine, where medical decisions and interventions are tailored to individual patients based on their genetic and biological risks for disease or predicted response to treatments. State-of-the-art medical care is certainly a big part of it, but personalized healthcare is the overall experience that is fueled by strong partnerships among patients, family members, all members of the care team, and other community partners as needed.

Personalized care emphasizes the active participation of patients and their families in the healthcare decision-making process as part of a cohesive strategy of healthcare services to help patients heal physically and emotionally.

Personalized healthcare responds to the physical, emotional, and social needs of each patient and may include complementary therapies such as massage, reiki, therapeutic touch, and pet therapy. Personalized healthcare incorporates the nurturing aspects of food. Nutrition is integral to healing, not only for good health but also for pleasure, comfort, and familiarity. The vital role of spirituality in caring for the whole person is also recognized, as are music and art, which can soothe the mind and feed the soul.

> Personalized care emphasizes the **active participation** of patients and their families in the healthcare decision-making process

This is not complicated or new age. In fact, simple things can make a big difference. Can patients and their loved ones choose healthy meals that best fit their tastes and schedule? Can patients and their loved ones receive spiritual care and support whenever they need it? Do patients and their loved ones have access to entertainment and diversions to help decrease stress and increase engagement?

Think Whole Person Healthcare in Omaha is a health-focused, physician-led primary care practice that views everyone as people with particular needs, wants, and dreams, not just as patients with symptoms and conditions. Their mission is reducing health costs by keeping patients who struggle with multiple ongoing conditions (such as diabetes, heart disease, and COPD) healthy and out of acute settings (the ER and hospital).

Their teams of doctors, pharmacists, nurses, and care coordinators help patients proactively manage their conditions to reduce suffering, improve clinical outcomes, lower costs, and enhance the experience of healthcare. They accomplish this by doing the simple tasks effectively—listening to patients and family caregivers, working to lower medication use and costs, helping to organize things for patients and family caregivers, and creating a plan with patients and family caregivers to ensure everyone gets the best out of life. And they do all of this in a beautiful, patient-friendly facility so customers can have the best experience possible.

In a similar vein, Apple and Amazon are aggressively embracing holistic care and focusing on wellness programs and prevention in their attempts to lower the cost of medical care for their employees. They're placing higher value on nurses, health coaches, nutritionists, fitness advisors, counselors, and over-the-counter remedies. They're investing more in clicks and virtual connectivity than in buildings or clinics. They're pricing their services simply and making awareness readily available. And they're defining success by improvements in employees' health status, as well as in reductions of procedures, tests, and admissions.

Demystify Healthcare

As healthcare has increased in scope and complexity, traditional healthcare settings became intimidating and confounding for many patients and their families. The physical size and arrangement of many hospitals is confusing, and the technologies that are often part of care settings can seem daunting even to medical providers.

In addition, the language used in healthcare can be bewildering for even the most sophisticated people, and more than that each entity may have a completely different meaning to the terms people think they understand. This can easily become too much for patients and their families who may be experiencing a life-changing event.

Medical staff need to take every opportunity to make patients and their families feel welcome, orient them to their room and the equipment/supplies that are present, let them know what's going on as well as what will be happening, and provide whatever ongoing information and assurances are necessary to meet their needs.

This process needs to be an open, two-way dialogue where patients and their family members feel free to ask any questions or raise any issues, and it needs to begin when the patient enters the facility and not end until the patient is discharged, in addition to any follow-up calls or appointments. It should also include easy access for patients to see and understand what's contained in their own medical record so they can actively participate in their own care and healing.

Here's a story from one of our colleagues that illustrates the imperative to ensure medical facilities are safe for patients and their guests as well as for staff members: "Without basic safety, nothing else matters. The facility was horrible in the women's day surgery area. In my observation room, the bed was sideways to the door and took all but about two feet of the width. Anyone who needed to reach my right side (where the IV was) had to go around the foot of the bed. There was a shelf with sharp corners just at head height right at the end of the bed. Every caregiver who went around the bed hit his or her head on that. One even opened a wound on his head! AND…the door knob to the room was installed upside down. People kept getting trapped in the room because they couldn't get the door open."

Our friend's experience illustrates the imperative to ensure medical facilities are safe for patients and their guests as well as for staff members. Without basic safety, nothing else matters.

Use Technology to Empower Patients

Rapidly improving technologies are already positioning inpatient and outpatient care for significant patient-centric disruption. The Department of Veterans Affairs (VA) has partnered with a tech company to develop a voice-activated virtual assistant that makes it easier for veterans to schedule appointments. Those appointments are then integrated with their health records and the VA's workflow.

Virtual assistants can also be used to collect demographic information, insurance details, and patient health history. Voice recognition technology exists to allow patients to dictate their information and have it automatically captured and loaded into their chart. These types of fundamental interactions between patients and technology will eliminate time-consuming hassles, wasteful paper-based documentation, and enable such data to be used immediately by medical providers. This doesn't even account for the potential of data mining and analysis of all the records.

The VA is in front of much of this by providing virtual assistants to patients. In essence, the VA has replaced 1950s-era call buttons with user-friendly technology that enables patients to find out many of the things they typically want to know (examples include "When will my doctor be here?" "What's for lunch?" "Do I have any dietary restrictions?" "Can I order a meal?"). Simple questions for which patients need answers can now be handled electronically rather than interrupting healthcare staff. But if a human touch is needed, virtual assistants can even be used to summon a nurse.

Further, interactive voice response systems such as Google Now, Siri, and others possess high-powered engines that can interact with unstructured data and fulfill requests at a highly accurate rate. It's not too far off when sick or injured people will be able to speak into a digital assistant at their home to find out whether they should head to an emergency room or to their primary care physician, depending on their condition and medical history.

Other medical providers are already leveraging digital assistants to enable their patients to perform a variety of tasks, including making hands-free calls to other people and allowing medical staff or family members to conduct drop-in visits with patients who agree to give such access. This is important for patients who need to be checked in on periodically.

Patients can also set up an electronic calendar for caregiver schedules. The technology can then check on staff schedules to see who is going to be on the next shift, set reminders for routine tasks such as taking medications, set up doctor appointments, answer patients' health-related queries, and generally stay on track with their treatment plan.

Make it Easy for Patients to Access Care

As we described earlier, transportation plays an essential role in quality of life. With respect to healthcare, barriers to transportation have a tremendous impact on people's health as well as the quality of care they receive.

So instead of building incredibly expensive parking garages for patients and employees, ride-hailing companies like Uber or Lyft can provide nonemergency transportation to/from health facilities. Both companies have healthcare offshoots and can eliminate transportation as a barrier to care. Consider a health system that subsidizes staff transportation to/from work to eliminate that hassle from their lives.

RECOMMENDED DISRUPTIVE INNOVATION #5
START A BEHAVIORAL REVOLUTION TO FOCUS ON HEALTH, NOT JUST SICK CARE

Unhealthy behaviors such as poor eating habits, lack of exercise, and smoking cost this country an estimated $1.5 billion each year in the treatment of preventable conditions such as heart disease, cancer, lung diseases, and diabetes, according to the 2017 *Annual Report of America's Health Rankings*. But as our healthcare system gains proficiency in treating chronic diseases, it is clear that Americans are struggling to modify behaviors that contribute to these diseases in the first place.

Despite the plethora of evidence buttressing the importance of prevention as a way to save lives and money, the majority of healthcare spending is directed toward treating illness.

Among the costliest and most preventable health conditions, chronic diseases (such as heart disease; cancer; lung diseases such as COPD, emphysema, and bronchitis; and diabetes) are directly linked with obesity and smoking, which are the two largest risk factors.

In fact, obesity is growing faster than any previous public health issue in the US. According to the most recent statistics, over 93 million American adults—nearly 40 percent of the adult population—are considered obese. It is estimated that obesity has added $344 billion to the nation's annual healthcare costs and accounts for more than 21 percent of total healthcare spending. Further, researchers found that obesity is the leading cause of preventable deaths and results in more life years lost—just over five years on average—than any other cause.

By focusing on treatment much more so than prevention, the healthcare industry is fighting the wrong battle. What should the industry do to include a stronger focus on prevention? What should the industry do to change people's behaviors to increase progress toward healthier lives and wellness? What should the industry do to change people's behaviors to reduce the burden of chronic diseases?

Remember our opening ideal future state in which people stay healthy and live a healthy lifestyle at home, at work, and in the community as you read the following recommendations:

» Every individual views staying healthy and living a healthy lifestyle as one of the most important things they can do.

» Parents model healthy behaviors for their children and instill in them a sense of the importance of staying healthy.

» Schools reinforce the message of health and well-being, and every student participates in daily physical education.

» Everyone walks more and spends more time engaged in physical activity than they do staring at a screen of any sort.

» Stand-up desks are ubiquitous at work and schools, and elevators are only used to go more than five floors.

» Memberships at gyms and fitness clubs are at an all-time high and are busy places most of the time.

» Salaries for fitness/health/strength coaches are comparable to those of other college-educated professions.

» Careers in healthcare—besides doctors and nurses—are more widely known, appreciated, and viewed as excellent occupational choices with above-average compensation.

Make the Health of Your Staff a Priority

Changing behaviors for an entire population is a daunting, if not impossible, challenge. But just like succeeding in other difficult undertakings, starting small and working from there can be an effective approach.

So why not begin your behavior change revolution by focusing on the people you work with every day—your staff members. Recall the high-tech disruptors (these are Amazon–Berkshire Hathaway–JP Morgan Chase, Apple, and Alphabet/Google) who are focusing exclusively on reducing healthcare costs by helping their own employees with better prevention and wellness. They are primarily thinking about employee health and join the 80 percent of employers who offer preventive and wellness services to their staff. They also recognize the role wellness can play in keeping their workforce healthy, engaged, and productive.

If your organization already has a wellness program for staff, consider how you can expand and enhance it to create a corporate culture of health. If not, consider starting an initiative. The key is to tailor the program to make the activities relevant for your employees, to address their wants (a survey) and needs (biometric data) and be inclusive. You can't just throw a smoking cessation program at a small percentage of employees who will never quit smoking and expect success. You can't just put a few treadmills into an empty office and call it good. Or offer to subsidize gym memberships.

Successful programs start with data gathering (surveys, insurance claims data, and just observation). You certainly don't want only healthy employees participating, and you want to extend participation to spouses and children to reinforce the importance home life can have on health and wellness.

Most corporate wellness programs recognize the physical component of health. Such efforts help employees learn about and make healthy choices regarding their bodies. These include increasing physical activity and exercise (in an environment where taking the stairs is the option of choice), increasing intake of nutritious foods like whole grains, fruits, and vegetables (and offering healthier and lower-cost choices in vending machines and cafeterias), and making private, third-party coaches available for employees who want to address smoking, weight loss, lack of sleep, addictions, financial problems, mental health challenges, and other major lifestyle change issues.

Specific interventions that enhance employees' physical health include biometric screenings, flu shots, opportunities for physical activity at work (and bosses that support the effort), nutrition education, as well as healthy snack choices and meals at the office.

The successful employee wellness programs also include elements to account for and connect other factors that impact people's wellness, happiness, and life. In addition to physical wellness, these other components include financial, emotional, and social wellness. To optimize a person's well-being, it is necessary for them to understand how the different components of wellness influence one another. For example, employees who are struggling with a financial issue are more likely to feel emotional and physical impacts as well. Also, when one aspect of wellness is lacking, it can be challenging for employees to be fully engaged with their work responsibilities.

In terms of financial wellness, many people have little understanding of basic financial principles and are thus unable to negotiate the financial landscape, manage financial risks effectively, and avoid financial pitfalls. According to one study by GreenPath Financial Wellness, 71 percent of employees say their top source of stress is personal finances. A study by the Society for Human Resource Management found that when people are stressed about their finances, both their physical health and productivity at work can be negatively impacted.

Earlier we mentioned efforts by Comcast to boost the financial literacy of their employees by creating and investing in a new company called Brightside, an online platform, to reduce employee financial stress. Including financial wellness as part of an overall workplace wellness program that helps employees become better educated and less worried about their finances will enable them to be happier and more engaged and thus less likely to miss work or suffer from health problems.

Organizations can integrate the financial component of wellness into their staff wellness program in several ways, including providing staff with access to financial advisors, retirement planning, investment advice, debt reduction and insurance planning, tuition reimbursement, and others. Any improvement in financial literacy will have a profound impact on employees, their ability to provide for their future, and their motivation at work.

71 percent of employees say their top source of stress is personal finances.

Emotional wellness is the ability to successfully handle life's stresses and adapt to change and challenging times. How people feel can affect their ability to carry out everyday activities, their relationships, and their overall mental health. Although more difficult to address in a work setting, it is crucial that employers support a healthy mental state and well-being. Without positive emotional well-being, employees will not be able to perform at their best while working.

Employers can assimilate the emotional component of wellness into their employee wellness program in a variety of ways, including stress management programs, meditation and mindfulness programs, deep breathing exercises, adequate paid time off, a robust employee assistance program, as well as emotional and mental health resources.

Finally, feeling like one has friends, social connections, and people they can confide in at work is an important determinant of overall satisfaction with a job and an employer as well as for overall happiness and well-being. Employees who do not feel connected with other people at work are more likely to be disengaged from their jobs and perform at lower levels than staff who do feel as if they are part of something unique and special.

Feelings of inclusion are part of an organizational culture. Organizations can include the social component of wellness into their staff wellness program in many ways by fostering team events, activities and outings, work-related celebrations, charitable campaigns, wellness challenges, book/reading clubs, and simply providing the space and opportunity for employees to socialize.

Wellness incentives come in all shapes and sizes, and employees respond to programs that are customized to their individual needs and goals. Draper Inc., Novartis, and GlaxoSmithKline are a few of the companies that offer personalized assistance by having wellness coaches meet individually with employees onsite to identify what they would like to change, discuss barriers that prevent them from changing, and then create an action plan to achieve what they want. Staff meet regularly with their coach to discuss goals, progress, and concerns. Such coaching empowers individuals and helps them feel valued.

Employees at Draper, for example, have access to a communal garden, a track, workout stations, table tennis, and volleyball courts. The company also has unique challenges with big rewards, including a yearlong step challenge whose most active participant is rewarded with a trip for two to Hawaii. Novartis offers subsidies for joining local sporting teams, health workshops on topics such as mindfulness and smoking cessation, and free health screenings. In addition, the company's cafeterias make the healthiest options on the menu the least expensive.

Wellness programs need to constantly evolve to remain relevant for employees and viable over time. A wide-ranging, sustained approach can pay off. Draper has seen improvements in employee health since it started tracking health data. Over five years, Draper has seen improved average values in a variety of employee health indicators, including BMI (body mass index, a measure of obesity)

> **Wellness programs need to constantly evolve to remain relevant for employees and viable over time.**

reduced by 6 percent, blood pressure down by 19 percent, glucose levels decreased by 1 percent, cholesterol levels down by 10 percent, and smoking cessation increased by 16 percent.

Each year there are more opportunities for new campaigns and incentives using social media as well as by capitalizing on the increasing number of people who are tracking their own health data. Although wellness programs are a positive step and have delivered clear results toward improved employee health, consistent behavioral change over time is needed to turn the tide on chronic diseases. In our view, the solution to better health relies on engaging and empowering individuals.

Provide Health-Wellness Coaches for Chronically Ill Patients

Healthy behaviors are not always the most important priority for individuals, and many people fail to live healthy lives. Many different motivators—such as managing time for work and family obligations, alleviating stress, or seeking pleasure—can compete with motives to pursue health.

As we mentioned earlier in this section, countless studies have shown that a few preventable behaviors such as poor diet, physical inactivity, tobacco use, and alcohol consumption place people at an increased risk for a variety of debilitating conditions (notably, type 2 diabetes, cardiovascular diseases such as heart attack, high blood pressure, and high cholesterol, stroke, COPD, some cancers, and premature death). Yet despite being so obvious, these unhealthy behaviors have become the leading causes of disease, premature death, and a dominant health issue of our time.

Rather than just prescribing treatments for the symptoms of chronic diseases, medical providers should do more to help patients reduce or eliminate their unhealthy behaviors that are causing the problems in the first place. One way to help the sickest, most needy, and most expensive patients is to incorporate a health-wellness coach into their overall care coordination team. Such health-wellness coaches can dive deeply into patients' own health and well-being to create personalized plans that implement realistic and sustainable changes to reduce patients' unhealthy behaviors so they can feel better every day.

Such health-wellness coaches often shift the focus away from behavioral-based outcomes—eat fewer refined carbohydrates, exercise more often, lose twenty pounds, for example—to a more narrative approach that allows patients to recognize the full story (such as a bad marriage or unruly kids or financial stress) underlying their behaviors so they can craft a new narrative with the types of outcomes they more deeply desire. Engaging patients in a coaching relationship actively engages them in a growth model of learning and healing and, when successful, can transform their health.

One approach to transforming population health is the Camden Coalition of Healthcare Providers (CCHP), a citywide coalition of hospitals, primary care providers, and community representatives that collaborate to deliver better healthcare to their most vulnerable citizens. They believe if they can improve care and reduce healthcare costs in Camden, NJ, it can be done for everyone, everywhere in America.

Coalition members share information through the Camden Health Information Exchange. With relevant, real-time data, their cross-disciplinary care teams connect quickly with people who have high rates of hospitalization and emergency room use and help them address their complex needs. Since 2002, the CCHP has demonstrated that human-centered, coordinated care, combined with the smart use of data, can improve patients' quality of care and reduce expensive, ineffective inpatient stays and emergency room visits. And that's better for everyone.

While healthcare providers may be compassionate, kind, and respectful of patients' needs and wishes and have the best interests of patients in mind, they often do not relate well to patients on a personal level. What's often missing is a layer of empathy that could spark patient behavior change. Health-wellness coaches can shift the traditionally paternalistic approach of care to one that is more in partnership with the patient. It involves listening differently to patients, rather than prescribing a fix. It involves listening to understand patients' experiences and finding openings for change. And it involves providing more timely feedback about and reinforcement of desired behaviors. It's not about making the patient fit into a prescriptive management approach, but instead about making that approach fit the patient.

> **What's often missing is a layer of empathy that could spark patient behavior change.**

Some areas of healthcare have used a coaching approach to achieve good patient outcomes. The CDC's Diabetes Prevention Program (DPP) is a good example. DPP does an excellent job of making the necessary resources available to patients (through healthcare providers, workplaces, community groups, schools, and churches) so they can identify their own health goals, determine the behaviors that will fit into their lifestyle, and guide patients in fulfilling their goals. Through regular coaching sessions and other patient engagement resources, the CDC has demonstrated that it is possible to cap diabetes in patients at risk for developing the disease.

Organizations like the Institute for Functional Medicine seek to understand how and why illness occurs and to teach forward-thinking medical care providers that medicine must shift from an acute-care approach to more effective prevention and chronic-disease management. They realize the future of medicine rests on addressing the root causes of our country's health problems and better understanding the complex interactions among lifestyle, genetics, and environment.

Partner to Build Healthy Communities

We already know the risk factors, and we already know what to do to help people live healthier and longer lives. We can make it easier for people to be physically active. We can make it easier for people to avoid tobacco. We can make it easier for people to have access to healthy and affordable food. We can make it easier for people to get recommended clinical preventive services and screenings. We can make it easier for people to receive routine dental care. We can make it easier for everyone to have access to high-quality healthcare when it's needed. We can make it easier for children to reach adulthood without facing potentially lifelong struggles with health issues. And we can make staying healthy and living a healthy lifestyle one of the most important tasks everyone can and wants to do.

"The power of community to create health is far greater than any physician, clinic, or hospital," according to Mark Hyman, MD, medical director at Cleveland Clinic's Center for Functional Medicine and the founder of the UltraWellness Center.

The healthcare industry needs to take the lead in acting on this knowledge. We can succeed by investing resources, using proven strategies, and creating a coalition with other sectors of the community (such as education, government, business, and social services) to improve health across our broader population. We have the strengths within our industry and our communities to help people live healthier and longer lives. Even identifying and focusing on one issue that needs to be addressed in a particular community can make a difference.

An example of such a community difference occurred in St. Louis. Many patients face significant social issues, such as homelessness, food insecurity, and unemployment. In many cases, these issues are more significant drivers of their health than clinical issues. Although hospitals and health systems have case management and social work experts available to direct these patients to social services, they often operate with limited information about what specific social services are available for individual patient needs. For example, a homeless diabetic patient may need access to housing options that provide refrigeration for insulin storage. Unfortunately, knowing which homeless shelters have an available bed and refrigeration facilities is often challenging.

In response to this need, the BJC/WUSM's Healthcare Innovation Lab is partnering with a company that has developed a common data platform that both the health system and social service organizations, such as homeless shelters, can use. The platform enables current and comprehensive accounting of available resources in the community and thus allows for tailored referrals and support for patients in need.

BJC's early experience with this platform suggests that it is not only helpful in coordinating efforts between the health system and social service organizations, but also allows for better coordination among social service organizations, such as homeless shelters and food pantries.

eTransX provides another example of community collaboration—in this case to address substance use disorders and the opioid epidemic. Research shows that it can take eight years, and four to five attempts at treatment, for the average person addicted to opioids to achieve one year of remission. But with the rise in the use of street drugs such as fentanyl, sobriety is becoming an increasingly risky proposition.

Nashville-based eTransX has taken on this challenge by offering a new software designed to facilitate coordination of diagnosis, treatment, and recovery services across the many stakeholders involved, including patients, patients' families, medical providers, care coordinators, peer recovery coaches, and government agencies.

While there is no single formula to create a healthy community, the key is collective action in which all the sectors— healthcare, local government, education, business, nonprofits, and other groups as well as individual citizens—work together for a common purpose. The guiding principle should be that communities must determine their preferred vision for the future based on the social, economic, environmental, and physical factors that influence the health of their people. As such, communities need to collectively determine their own needs and create action plans to improve residents' quality of life based on the community's specific needs, characteristics, and assets.

> ...communities must determine their preferred **vision for the future** based on the social, economic, environmental, and physical factors that influence the health of their people.

The greatest impact comes when we make the healthy choice the default choice, and part of the normal course of everyday life. Healthy communities are based on five strategies that build on a community's existing capacity to improve community health and well-being: community involvement, political commitment, healthy public policy, multisector collaboration, and asset-based community development.

Another example of community intervention is Hennepin Medical Center in Minneapolis, which decided that to reduce costs it should look at all the ways it was spending money. After digging into the data, they discovered that forty-two people in a twelve-month period cost the hospital nearly $10 million. Someone at the discussion flippantly remarked, "For this kind of money we could buy them all a condo and limo."

That was never going to happen, but everyone understood the point that the hospital was spending an average of $238,095 for each of these people and something needed to be done. The next step was to dig into their care and determine if they were placed appropriately, provided care at the appropriate healthcare provider skill level, and so forth. As is often the case, many of these people didn't really need a hospital. Instead they required other support from the community such as housing, counseling, food, welfare, and other social services.

One patient was admitted to the hospital twenty-eight times over a twelve-month period. Diagnosis? Sleeping under a bridge in weather that was often below zero, undernourished, and in need of psychiatric care. Deciding to sleep in a cardboard box or getting admitted to a warm hospital with a comfortable bed, three meals, and nurses to care for him wasn't a tough call and no one could blame him. However, the hospital was not where he needed to be.

The hospital worked with social services to get him and several of the other high utilizers the help they really needed. By addressing the root causes of these patients' issues, their quality of life was enhanced and the cost of providing care to the community was significantly reduced.

There are numerous examples of healthy community initiatives across the country. Here are just a few of them.

In collaboration with state government, state universities, and healthy community organizations, Blue Cross Blue Shield of Michigan instituted a statewide program to help school children learn about good nutrition and get more exercise. The intent was to reduce the impact obesity has on children's health and school performance by creating supportive school environments through healthy eating and physical activity.

Focusing on children in grades K-12, this program provides the knowledge and helps establish the behaviors necessary for a healthy lifestyle by educating students on nutrition and physical activity through classroom and gym lessons, creating a supportive environment that makes healthy choices easy, encouraging students to practice lessons learned in the classroom, providing opportunities for physical activity, and increasing access to healthy food and beverages.

Michigan's healthy communities initiative has demonstrated measurable impact on improving the health of children, including a significant reduction in obesity, 40 percent more fruit and vegetables consumed than the national average, 700-step increase per day, thirty-five additional minutes per week of moderate to vigorous physical activity, nineteen minutes less of screen and video time per day, and 74 percent of students report that it was easier to pay attention in class.

In New York City the people recognize that a community's health isn't limited to access to medical care. Physical and mental health are critical elements for improving social well-being, and vibrant public spaces are essential community resources where people can come together to play, learn, grow food, exercise, and relax. Yet many poor neighborhoods have historically been neglected from public investment in open spaces and playgrounds. These same communities often report high rates of crime and equally high rates of obesity and diabetes.

NYC's healthy community initiative marshals local, public, and private partners to address those inequities and improve community health outcomes in twelve neighborhoods across all five boroughs by improving opportunities for physical activity, increasing access to nutritious and affordable food, and promoting public safety.

Johns Hopkins Medicine is leading healthy community efforts in Baltimore through a number of programs focused on different aspects of the city. As parents, grandparents, and caring adults, the staff at Johns Hopkins Medicine want the next generation to be happy and healthy, so they have created several programs to teach children about the importance of healthy eating decisions and learning new skills for a future in the workplace.

BLocal, a consortium of Baltimore-area businesses has joined forces to expand existing programs or launch new ones to build, hire, invest, and buy locally. Taken together, BLocal commitments will infuse at least $69 million into local and minority-owned, women-owned, and disadvantaged businesses over the next three years.

The healthy community initiative also includes an innovative nutrition education program available to elementary schools in southeastern Baltimore City and Baltimore County, a youth community program that provides summer internships, scholarships, mentorship, and shadowing opportunities to students in Baltimore City, and the CARES Summer in the Lab enables undergraduate and high school interns to spend the summer at Johns Hopkins Medicine exploring different fields of research. These and other programs connect resources and people to develop future leaders and build a stronger Baltimore.

These are just a few successful initiatives that are making healthy choices easier, and they are starting to take root around the country. In San Francisco, 44,000 children now have access to safe recreational space because public school playgrounds are now open during nonschool hours.

In Broward County, Florida, nearly 700,000 residents can increase their level of physical activity because their community is improving the safety and accessibility of walking, riding bikes, and using public transportation. Improvements in community health can even come from simple measures that focus clinical attention on problem areas. These include effective use of electronic health records to identify and track the progress of patients who need support, team-based care, the use of protocols, and prompt data feedback.

Changing behaviors is never easy. But tens of thousands of preventable deaths occur each year because we fail to act. The healthcare industry owes it to the American people to do better. As TV's doctor, Mehmet Oz, MD, a cardiothoracic surgeon, observed, "True health care reform cannot happen in Washington. It has to happen in our kitchens, in our homes, in our communities. All health care is personal."

At the end of the day, it is people's small, everyday behaviors and actions that determine our health. We need to take care of ourselves day in and day out by making smart, healthy choices. We need to change how we live our lives. Fortunately, small changes in our diets and increased physical activity can go a long way to helping people stay healthy as well as reducing the risk factors for chronic diseases. The healthcare industry and medical providers are perfectly positioned to lead a behavioral revolution that helps people be smarter about what they do and what they eat.

> Changing behaviors is never easy. But tens of thousands of preventable deaths occur each year because **we fail to act.**

CHAPTER TAKEAWAYS

There is a growing state of consumer agitation with healthcare, a groundswell of employers who are taking a more activist role in the health of their employees, and disruptive innovators who see opportunity and are doing something about it. These forces are poised to drive a revolution in healthcare.

In this chapter we described what healthcare leaders can (and should) do right now to disrupt their organizations for the sake of long-term relevance and survival. These were ideas about how to position the industry to be competitive in the future, and include:

» Create pricing transparency to drive affordable care and real choice.

» Provide easy access to care where and when consumers want it.

» Turn providers into health partners.

» Make clinical settings warm and friendly places to heal (and to work).

» Start a behavioral revolution to make people healthier.

Nearly everyone recognizes that prevailing business models in healthcare must profoundly change. A wide range of industries—retail, transportation, manufacturing, entertainment and media, and grocery—have already been deeply affected. No industry or organization, including healthcare, can afford to ignore the threat. Yet most healthcare organizations are not moving fast enough to meet this challenge. We believe the power of disruptive innovation and free-market forces must be unleashed to shift everyone's focus from sick care to healthcare.

3

How Healthcare Can Medicate Itself: A Big, Bittersweet Dose of **Disruption**

IT MUST BE CONSIDERED THAT THERE IS NOTHING MORE DIFFICULT TO CARRY OUT NOR MORE DOUBTFUL OF SUCCESS NOR MORE DANGEROUS TO HANDLE THAN TO INITIATE A NEW ORDER OF THINGS.

—*Niccolò Machiavelli (1469–1527)*

Up to this point, we have described the disruptive threats confronting the healthcare industry and shared key actions that should be undertaken in the short term to transform healthcare organizations in ways that meet the evolving consumer demands. These are all ideas about what can be done to improve the delivery of healthcare and to be competitive in the future healthcare marketplace.

Now, let's talk about how to be disruptive and bring about meaningful change.

The challenge is to engage in disruptive innovation or be disrupted by someone else, either inside or outside the industry. For incumbents in any industry, disruptive innovation is particularly hard. In healthcare, many will struggle to see the possibilities. Some will admit that they will have to be dragged from the fee-for-service environment into at-risk contracts. Others will flirt with disruptive innovation, giving it lip service, but will not make substantive changes. And a few will recognize the imperative to change significantly, but won't have a clue where or how to start. This is one of our main reasons for writing this book.

Of course, some may consider whether they want to change at all. As management consultant W. Edwards Deming said, "It is not necessary to change. Survival is not mandatory."

As you read this chapter on creating a culture of disruption in healthcare organizations, keep in mind our ideal future state:

» Medical errors have been reduced to zero, and similar to aircraft crashes, any that occur are studied and the findings widely published so that the same error is never made twice.

» Everyone in healthcare is trained in improvement and innovation, and their mindset is consumer-focused improvement, rapid cycle testing of new ideas, and abandonment of any practice that is not evidence-based and achieving results.

» A culture of asking questions and continuous learning pervades healthcare organizations.

» The entire healthcare industry has become a source of rapid cycle testing of new ideas, and a place where innovation smoothly follows more innovation.

BARRIERS TO DISRUPTING HEALTHCARE

Why is it so difficult for established organizations to innovate their business models and practices? Why is it such a challenge to step away from what seems to be working and try something different? What would allow organizations to innovate more deeply and broadly? What approach would allow established organizations to overturn the underlying premises of their industries before others do?

Our work across the healthcare industry suggests that established organizations *can* disrupt traditional ways of doing business. They can disrupt themselves in a variety of ways provided they understand and master the barriers that stand in their way. The first barrier to overcome is reframing your underlying beliefs regarding value creation.

Barrier #1: Underlying Beliefs

Every industry is built around long-standing, often implicit beliefs about how to serve customers and to make money. In ground transportation, for example, it's believed that on-time delivery and accuracy are key indicators of success. In commercial aviation, it's capacity (how full the planes are) and money made per mile flown. Time necessary to obtain approval from the FDA is fundamental for pharmaceutical companies. For content delivery companies like Netflix, customer growth and retention define success. For social media, the number of hits drives profitability. And so on.

These governing beliefs reflect widely shared and often unspoken notions about customers and customer preferences and competitors and the impact of technology, regulations, and cost drivers. These underlying beliefs strongly influence organizational structures to deliver products and services, yet also constrain people's thinking and ability to disrupt themselves.

Everyone in healthcare will tell you the fundamental, underlying belief is that patients come first.

We question if the underlying belief isn't more accurately that "we need to *say* the patient comes first" while little we actually do reflects that. The first thing many receptionists say to you upon arrival in the doctor's office is "Insurance?" It's telling that they don't want to know our names and how we are doing.

The problem is that very little in the current system supports the premise that patients come first. The very foundation of healthcare is no longer the consumer/patient, but rather hospitals, insurers, doctors, and drug manufacturers. Examples of this are numerous and begin with staffing and scheduling at most hospitals and clinics, which suggests an eight-to-five Monday through Friday set-up rather than the 24/7 operation everyone professes to have.

> The problem is that very little in the current system supports the premise that **patients come first.**

If you're thinking, "wait a minute, hospitals *are* open 24/7," ask yourself the following questions: How many nonclinical staff are scheduled during the days versus the nights? How many medical providers are present during the days versus the nights? How many procedures are performed during the days versus the nights? How many patients are discharged during the day versus at night?

Your answers will vividly illustrate that healthcare organizations are anything but 24/7 operations. Just because the lights are still on and a few staff are present doesn't mean the organization is functioning. Such bank-like hours are done for the convenience of the administrators, providers, and staff, not for patients and their families. Try finding a doctor in the evenings or on weekends. It's small wonder why ERs around the country are packed with nonemergent cases.

We can pretty much assure you that disruptive companies will find a way to move care in time and space so that consumers are able to access care whenever and wherever it is convenient for them. That is, they will make care truly available 24/7, and they will move the care closer to the customer, including into consumers' homes.

As another example, consider the 340b Drug Program that provides rebates to hospitals, but does absolutely nothing to reduce the cost of prescription medications to consumers, who don't see a penny of any savings or rebates. The outrageous price of prescription medications is a glaring example of where patients don't come first.

Former FDA Administrator Scott Gottlieb, MD, has even called contracts between pharmaceutical companies and insurers "kabuki drug-pricing constructs" because they are so convoluted and profit the industry at the expense of consumers.

Another example is hospital and clinic billing, where the primary customer is the insurer. At best, patients are secondary, and there is absolutely no incentive to reduce costs to consumers or—unlike a roofer, mechanic, barber, CPA, attorney, or any other profession— make it clear exactly how much patients will be charged prior to providing care. There are so many other examples of patients not coming first that it would be impossible to list them all.

A corollary of patients not really coming first, which is rarely spoken but has been in place for a long time, is that it is a privilege for patients to get to come and receive our wonderful care. Rarely do providers apologize or explain themselves when they make patients wait for an hour (beyond their appointment time) for the privilege of seeing them. That their time is more valuable than patients' is a given.

In all of our years, neither of us has ever had a healthcare provider at a hospital or doctor's office thank us for coming to their place of business. The assumption is that patients come to providers; we don't go after them in some competitive marketplace. This rather passive approach to doing business, which served healthcare adequately in the past, will face an increasingly bleak future. There is an excellent book titled

The Patient Will See You Now by Dr. Eric Topol. The title alone implies this physician has a different set of underlying assumptions about how providers and patients should think and behave.

A final underlying and unspoken belief is that healthcare exists to diagnose symptoms and treat sickness, rather than prevent illness in the first place. This is completely understandable in a fee-for-service environment because that is basically all healthcare providers get paid to do. The reality is that a huge amount of cost is incurred in the healthcare system because sickness is not prevented.

Terry was on the executive team in a California safety net hospital. He remembers asking physicians in the emergency department, "Are we seeing a lot of patients in the ED that don't need to be seen in an ED?" The answer from the physicians was, "No, for the most part the people we see are sick enough to merit being in the emergency department. However, many of them should have never become that sick in the first place. If they had received proper primary care or any primary care at all, they would have never become so sick that a visit to the ED was needed."

It's appropriate to note that "there are more than 9,000 billing codes for individual procedures and units of care," according to Clayton Christensen, author of *The Innovator's Prescription: A Disruptive Solution for Health Care.* "But there is not a single billing code for patient adherence or improvement, or for helping patients stay well."

These are just a few examples of underlying assumptions that will have to be challenged and rethought. It is our set of underlying assumptions that drives our behavior and often constrains our ability to consider different possibilities. To change behavior permanently without changing underlying assumptions is virtually impossible.

Barrier #2: Not Understanding Customers

Innovation does not necessarily mean coming up with the latest and greatest. It has nothing to do with outdoing competitors with bigger and better. Innovation comes directly from a deep understanding of one's customers.

Disruptive innovation does more than empower customers. It creates entirely new customer segments, with different needs and expectations. One of the most obvious transformations in the current healthcare landscape is the growing involvement of people in their own care. Consumers have become more informed and engaged with their own health and decisions regarding healthcare.

Combined with the fact that consumers are responsible for an increasing share of their healthcare costs, people are beginning to change the way they make healthcare decisions. For many types of care, they are acting more like traditional consumers who compare prices to shop around for the best deal. This phenomenon will continue to spread, with business model implications for hospitals, physicians, and the broader healthcare industrial complex.

This story from one of our friends illustrates how hospitals don't really understand their customers: "I love my surgeon, but the hospital is a nightmare. My husband was wild with irritation at their poor family communication process. The pre-op room had been a mother/baby room but was now women's surgery. The outdated whiteboard—'Your baby's nurse today'—didn't bother me, but what if a woman who hoped to have more children was in for a hysterectomy? There was no chair for my husband in the pre-op area. The nurse doing the pre-op was interrupted three times while she was trying to give me my meds. Can you say medication error? I watched her like a hawk to make sure she scanned everything just before I took it. For my pre-op assessment the week before, I had to see the surgeon in one part of town and the anesthesia NP thirty minutes away an hour later."

But what do consumers really want? A 2018 study by the Urgent Care Association of America (UCAA) found that consumers value three things with respect to their healthcare. First and most fundamentally, consumers want to know what the price of something is if they buy it from vendor A compared to vendor B. Is this not true for the items you and your family purchase?

Transparency is what everyone wants for any product or service, and it's a given in every other industry except healthcare. Even the airlines publish their fares, although they may change from one minute to the next. As consumers become more responsible for paying the fees for healthcare services, they will need (and they deserve to have) reliable, clear, and accessible pricing in advance.

> To remain competitive, the visibility of healthcare pricing and other information consumers require for assessing value must be **radically improved.**

To remain competitive, the visibility of healthcare pricing and other information consumers require for assessing value must be radically improved. It must become much more transparent, accessible, and defensible. Medical providers should go beyond mere compliance with the Centers for Medicare & Medicaid Services rule that requires hospitals to post their charge masters online.

We said this in a previous section but will repeat it here because it is critical. Providers should determine what they need to charge to remain profitable (based on their actual costs), keep it simple, and empower patients with cost and quality information. Providers need to create the type of value-based system and more transparent pricing that Amazon, Boeing, Cisco, Comcast, Disney, and Walmart all provide to their customers, are already looking for from healthcare, and that other large employers (and eventually consumers) will soon be demanding.

Besides visibility of costs, what else do consumers want from the healthcare system? The second major thing people want is *ease of access*. Consumers are demanding more convenient options for their healthcare needs. Consumers want the same on-demand model for healthcare that they have in the rest of their lives. Let's face it, people can sell homes, manage investment portfolios, consult legal experts, and do many more activities with their phones. Is it not surprising that patient behavior is changing, and that consumers are no longer willing to wait a week (or even days) to see a doctor?

It used to be accepted as gospel that primary care physicians (PCPs) were the first step for finding care. The 2018 UCAA study found that consumers are turning to convenient care, urgent care, and retail clinics at a rate of approximately 170 million visits per year. Their study also found that even when a consumer has a PCP, less than half of Americans use their PCP as the first step in finding care.

For people under the age of forty-five, this drops to 36 percent. There was also a significant gap between the need for care and the availability of providers. After "needed same-day attention," survey respondents selected "convenient location and time" as their second biggest reason for visiting a convenient/urgent care clinic.

Finally, consumers want the *ease of booking online*. The 2018 UCAA study found that consumers are not benefiting from the advances in healthcare technology as much as the industry believes. The reality is that consumers' basic needs are still unmet, and the top high-tech products requested by consumers are those that provide basic control and convenience.

The UCAA survey asked people what kind of healthcare technology would most meaningfully improve their experience in healthcare. Easy online and mobile booking—something widely available in many other industries for over a decade—was the top technology requested by survey respondents. In fact, 67 percent of respondents indicated this as their most important, and notably those aged forty-five to sixty requested it the most.

The technology that enables consumers to find the right healthcare provider and make an appointment online already exists. Zocdoc, an online medical care appointment booking service, provides free medical care search capabilities for consumers by integrating information about medical practices and physicians' individual schedules.

Finding the right healthcare provider and making an appointment is as simple as reading reviews and making a reservation—as many people have routinely been doing for restaurants, yoga studios, or hair salons for some time. With Zocdoc, consumers can read reviews of physicians, instantly make appointments, fill out paperwork before the visit, and receive reminders for checkups and other health-related items, all from the online service.

When you consider the gap between what consumers really want (that is, price transparency, ease of access, and ability to book online) and what the current healthcare system delivers, it is bewildering.

> While nearly every other industry has been redefined through **relentless focus** on meeting or exceeding the evolving consumer needs...healthcare lags far behind.

While nearly every other industry has been redefined through relentless focus on meeting or exceeding the evolving consumer needs and desires, healthcare lags far behind.

Empowered and emboldened consumers demanding that healthcare operate more like every other business will be a force that pushes the healthcare industry to provide significantly more visibility regarding cost and coverage, technology that enables ease of access, and providers who are willing to deliver care on patients' schedules rather than the other way around.

Barrier #3: Organizational (and Industry) Inertia

Think about the proud history of a large organization you are familiar with. We're pretty sure it didn't start out as the large, complicated enterprise it now is. In fact, if you dig deeply enough, you'll find that every organization begins as a start-up with an idea to meet some known or unknown consumer need. Typically, one, two, or a few people come together to solve a problem by producing something or creating a service that could be delivered to consumers. Many of today's large health systems started exactly this way.

In the early days, the founders' vision is clear and widely shared; everyone is focused on doing whatever it takes to serve customers; and overhead costs are relatively low. However, as an organization starts to grow, specialization begins to happen. In addition to specialties related to producing products or delivering services, administrative roles become necessary to run the business and to support those who are serving customers. As an organization continues to grow, staff are added and systems and structures are put into place to help manage the work production, service delivery, as well as the people.

Over time a variety of factors help shape an organization's culture. These include the founders' vision, values, preferences, and assumptions, the demands of the industry and its customers, as well as the ideas, customs, and social behaviors of people who work there. Culture is further molded and maintained by the various systems and structures that have been put into place as the organization matures. These include systems for recruitment and selection, new employee onboarding, staff development, performance evaluation, and reward systems—the combination of which make every organization distinct.

Contemporary healthcare organizations are composed of business units (such as service lines, departments, or clinics) that are designed to deliver on a value proposition. They include people, equipment, supplies, information, and processes. They are connected to upstream suppliers and downstream customers. Internal support departments support them. And they run most efficiently when standard work is in place and adhered to.

The unspoken job of leaders and staff is to protect the status quo and maybe to improve it incrementally when needed and as time permits. Any talk of changing an existing business unit in any major way is resisted (both subtly and overtly) by the status quo and is difficult to envision within the confines of the existing management systems and structures.

As we see it, one way to think of existing organizations is that they are living organisms with built-in antibodies that will destroy any outside ideas threatening to disrupt the status quo.

Change efforts frequently fail to address the underlying beliefs that constrain organizations' current mode of creating value, nor do they deal with the underlying culture of the organization. As a result, organizations (and entire industries) often get stuck by playing it safe. Their default form of innovation becomes improving what they already do, and changes become more incremental as organizations try to manage risks and maintain stability.

The status quo in the healthcare system is formidable. For the past thirty-plus years, the established players in the US healthcare industry have fared well. Annual spending for healthcare has routinely increased a few percentage points above inflation and overall economic growth; existing organizations have become bigger and stronger; the industry as a whole has outperformed the broader stock market over many longitudinal periods; and industry earnings tend to delight market analysts and fill shareholder pockets.

In addition, the industry has avoided being commoditized by stressing the complexity of medical care and emphasizing the challenges of regulatory compliance. Healthcare is comfortable with medical and technical innovation, but like many industries, it pushes hard against disruptors who dare to disturb the status quo. Sustaining innovations in the form of new drugs, devices, algorithms, payment schemes, consolidation, and regulatory compliance are the industry's standard fare. Who within the industry would want to change this? Anyone who dares disrupt this status quo to create competition or fundamentally alter how healthcare does things is largely unwelcome.

Barrier #4: Denial

Denial is a natural part of human nature that is closely related to the survival instinct. As a result, there is a tendency toward denial inherent in many organizations. Some would even say denial is endemic to management. But why is denial so prevalent?

First, denial typically happens over time as small parts of a pattern of behavior rather than a large, isolated event. So many people don't notice it or realize they are doing it. Second, denial is often easier, safer, and more comfortable than confronting a problem, a poor decision, or a failing strategy. Finally, denial can be beneficial, especially in the short term. As Elisabeth Kübler-Ross's stages of grief suggest, denial is the first step of the change process. It is natural and necessary and can help buy time to figure out how best to change.

The danger of denial lies in what is done about it. If alternatives are actively sought and if organizational capacities and resources are tapped, positive changes can occur and good outcomes can happen. However, if people stick their heads in the sand and do nothing, or if people work harder doing the old, outdated tasks they have always done, success is less likely. Often old products and services are just changed somewhat when they ought to be discarded altogether. Building slide rules with teakwood and pearl inlay won't help you sell any more in a world of smartphones.

Unfortunately, research abounds showing that people under stress tend to revert to behavior they are familiar with. This is true of organizational behavior as well. It explains why healthcare leaders sometimes pursue initiatives that are largely unnecessary, ineffective, or dangerous to their organization's future. Here are some examples:

» Thinking and acting like fee-for-service is here to stay

» Building more hospital beds than are needed

» Ignoring the opportunity to partner with companies in their communities by failing to ask what they need from healthcare and working hard to accommodate them

» Not engaging physicians in developing strategy for the future

» Considering mergers to create a monopoly without reducing cost to the payer (this has been done in most other industries that have been disrupted, and it never works long term)

» Thinking that the commodity care they grossly overcharge for in the hospital will not soon be offered outside the hospital at a third of the cost

» Thinking technology will magically save them from the onslaught to come

» Remaining in their historically passive mode believing customers love them so much they will always come back

» Failing to harness the brainpower of all of their staff (who could blossom into an army of problem solvers and innovators if they were ensconced in a culture that values experimentation and learning)

Some will adapt, but many will continue to do only what they already know how to and are comfortable with.

Lack of knowledge of the disruptive process—or thinking "it won't happen here"—has caused many organizations in a variety of industries to fail to engage before it was too late. Additionally, organizations attempting changes that are too large often fail. This is in part because they don't understand change management principles or they underestimate the effort required. For many, change is associated with loss or fear of being unable to operate in a new system. So the natural defensive response is to resist and sabotage.

One final point. Time is of the essence. It is easy to underestimate the speed of revolutions. It is often the case that change moves very slowly until the point at which it moves incredibly fast. In assessing the cost-benefit and risk of investments, we often make comparisons in the context of a world similar to today's circumstances. The more meaningful comparison, however, is against the environment that will exist in the future, which could be radically different. The market potential of a disruptive opportunity may seem insignificant relative to the size of your business today, but that calculus could be markedly different in a disrupted environment, where the share of the traditional offering has shrunk dramatically.

> **Time is of the essence. It is easy to underestimate the speed of revolutions.**

Barrier #5: Faulty Strategy–Focus Only on Higher Margin Products and Services

A final barrier to internal innovation occurs when an organization is losing market share, but only at lower levels with low margins. Strategically, it doesn't make sense to focus on the lower end of the market when the higher, more expensive end produces better margins.

According to noted innovation expert Clayton Christensen, new entrants can prove disruptive by beginning to target those overlooked segments and gain a foothold by delivering more suitable low-end functionality at a lower price. Incumbents chasing higher profitability in more demanding segments tend not to respond vigorously. But once established at the low end, new entrants then move upmarket, delivering the performance that existing organizations' mainstream customers require, while preserving the advantages that drove their early success. When mainstream customers start adopting the entrants' offerings in volume, disruption has occurred.

When Toyota entered the US market in 1968 with the unassuming Corolla, GM, Ford, and Chrysler did not see them as a threat. Toyota started the no frills Corolla with a ninety-inch wheelbase and a sixty-horsepower engine. Known as The Big Three at the time, GM, Ford, and Chrysler didn't bother to take Toyota seriously. Toyota was entering the lower end of the market, which equated to lower margins that did not make sense for the big three American companies to pursue because larger vehicles were where the larger profits were.

Over the decades Toyota progressed in size and quality until they launched the Lexus. In the process, The Big Three lost an embarrassing amount of market share, which they have never recovered.

Similarly, Digital Equipment Corporation (DEC) made huge mainframe computers, which were very expensive and required deep expertise to make. The business model required gross profits of 60 percent just to cover the inherent overhead. The personal computer disrupted this industry by making computing so affordable and accessible that millions could purchase and use computers.

DEC continued to pursue the high end of the market, and when it eventually tried to commercialize the personal computer, it did so from within its existing business model, which simply could not make money if the computers were priced below $50,000.

In contrast, IBM established a separate business unit that focused on personal computers. IBM deliberately kept this unit physically and organizationally separated from its mainframe and minicomputer business units. In its PC business model, IBM could make money with low margins, low overhead costs, and high unit sales volumes. By coupling the technological enablers that both DEC and IBM had with a new business model that only IBM had, IBM transformed the computing industry and much of the world with it, while DEC was swept away.

In healthcare, Belle Cares is a company causing disruption by doing low-end yet necessary services very well. Belle Cares provides foot and nail care in the home or retirement community or wherever needed by patients. Many elderly people need monthly care for their neuropathy, poor circulation, pain, or whatever else ails their feet. Many simply find it too difficult to make it to the podiatrist's office on a monthly basis.

So Belle Cares sends highly trained technicians who have caring hearts and warm personalities to the patients' homes. At the end of the visit, technicians ask patients when they would like another appointment so the patient doesn't have to bother with calling or going online to make it themselves. Patients grow attached to their technicians, and the technicians to their patients. Belle Cares is now disrupting the higher end portion of podiatrists' practices. This is a classic example of disruptive innovation and of making a product or service easy to use and more accessible.

Dealing with barriers to transforming your organization is humbling and difficult, but necessary.

MAKING DISRUPTION A
REALITY IN HEALTHCARE

Countless market-changing disruptions are in the works for healthcare. They are necessary, they are overdue, and because of employer and consumer pressure, they will happen. We've described a few of them and provided our thoughts about *what* healthcare leaders should do now to enable the survival of their organizations and ensure they are positioned for the future. As Charles Darwin observed, "It is not the strongest of the species that survives, nor the most intelligent, but the one most responsive to change."

This section addresses *how* leaders can adjust their organization and build its capabilities around long-term innovation to remain relevant, stay in business, and thrive into the future. And for the eternal optimists among us, we discuss how leaders can make healthcare better, more holistic and comprehensive, more human, and even something that approaches elegance.

Because of the aforementioned barriers, most organizations do not disrupt themselves very well. Some think it is impossible. We know it is possible, though difficult, and have seen examples where it is happening within healthcare.

A few healthcare organizations are innovating in deliberate, strategic ways (examples include Cedars Sinai, Cleveland Clinic, Denver Health, Geisinger, Johns Hopkins, Mayo Clinic, and several others). We will examine what they're doing, but also cast our net to other industries to glean what we can learn from them. Further, we will explore structures, activities, and tools that might be helpful as leaders embark on this journey of exploration, discovery, and the challenges required to create a new healthcare marketplace.

For any organization to disrupt itself, strong and unwavering support from senior leaders is imperative. Leaders must be willing to embrace failures and encourage learning from them. In addition, *all* efforts must be connected with strategy and prioritized as key initiatives so they do not get pushed aside by something more urgent but less important. And when a decision is made to move forward, it is imperative that the efforts not be institutionalized and thereby subjected to the organizational antibodies that would sabotage the changes required. Strong leadership at all levels is required to create the space for innovation, and to protect the innovators as well as the innovation process.

Eliminate Non-Value Adding Activities

First and foremost, after the decision is made to move in this direction, we recommend leaders begin by critically evaluating all initiatives throughout their organization and aggressively sunsetting as many as they can. The discipline is to stop any project, initiative, or activity that does not add value to customers and patients.

To get started, leaders, providers, and staff must ask themselves these questions:

» What is the reason we do this, in this way, in the first place?

» Would customers/patients think this activity is necessary?

» Would customers/patients be willing to pay for this? Does it add value?

» If we were at risk financially, would we continue to do this?

Sound strange? Not at all. A big problem in many organizations is that leaders continue to pile on new activities, projects, committees, task forces, metrics, procedures, policies, meetings, and so forth, endlessly. This is especially true around annual planning time. For some reason, it rarely occurs to leaders to prune back what they have everyone working on, to take things off their plates, and to stop engaging in activities that don't support the organiza-tion's strategy. The opportunity cost of this practice is immense.

Pruning a tree actually makes it stronger and more capable of producing fruit. Failing to do so weakens it, dissipating its limited resources. The same is true of any organization (especially healthcare), no matter how impressive their pedigree.

If leaders prune vigorously throughout the organization, we predict the following outcomes will happen:

» They will find more waste than they ever imagined.

» They will discover underlying assumptions and behav-iors that are outdated, unnecessary, and irrelevant.

» They will discover that executives, managers, provid-ers, and staff will appreciate them for showing respect for their challenges.

» Many will become energized and freed up to work on projects that are truly most important and will be happy to do so (no one wants to do meaningless work).

» Medical providers might have more time to actually pursue their calling—which is typically why they chose to work in healthcare in the first place.

Try it. It has worked wonders for those who have embraced it, and we know it can make a dramatic difference for healthcare organizations.

Enhance Your Current Improvement Activity

We also suggest a heavy dose of efficiency innovation. Remember, we said efficiency innovation is about eliminating waste, reducing cost, and improving quality. Many organizations have been doing this, and the process is still necessary. There is still huge waste in every healthcare organization. Whatever cannot be discarded should be simplified. Handoffs should be reduced, redundancies eliminated, and unnecessary steps removed. How sub-businesses, service lines, and departments are designed should be critically examined, as should where they are placed and how the support areas work. Does everyone know they have customers—internal or external—and do they know what their customers need? Does the system talk to itself?

Understand how things are communicated. Question every rule, every policy, and every step. Healthcare leaders should ask frontline staff to simplify their work to make it easier. They will have ideas, but leadership must go to where the work is being done and ask. Many staff ideas will be excellent. If leaders will go to the front lines, listen, encourage experimentation, and make it safe to fail fast and learn quickly, such action will reduce the need for many of the meetings executives sit through all day, every day. It will change the culture.

Next, healthcare leaders should ask about their organization's capacity for rapid improvement:

» Do they have an operational excellence, performance improvement, or lean department? If so, how is that functioning?

» Are they facilitating rapid improvement events?

» Are they training and coaching others to increase the organization's capacity for rapid improvement at all levels?

» Are they teaching and coaching problem-solving skills?

» Does the organization have an army of problem solvers who are well-versed in improvement tools and methods?

» Are standard work and visual management in place and in use throughout the organization?

» Have leaders created an environment that supports continual, rapid improvement?

» Have leaders created an environment that supports robust daily management?

We've consulted with numerous hospitals across the country for decades. Very few have all of these elements in place. To take it a step further, leaders can be asked these questions:

» Does your organization have hundreds of experiments in play all of the time (like Amazon)?

» Are your improvement teams, providers, and staff brainstorming ideas that will make things work ten times better (not just 10 percent) like Google does?

» Do they then turn around and test their ideas within the next day or two?

» How good is everyone at managing rapid change?

Amazon, Google, and many others are coming to disrupt healthcare. They are fed up. They think the healthcare industry's ways of doing business are outdated and far too costly. They don't care about the industry's underlying belief system. They don't think healthcare is effectively managed. They are smart, quick, savvy, and, in some cases, ruthless. It behooves healthcare leaders to put efficiency and sustaining improvement activity on steroids while they are initiating disruptive innovation. All three are necessary.

Commit to Learning Everything about Disruptive Innovation (including the Coming Threats and Opportunities)

Terry once heard a guest minister at a Baptist church in Dallas say, "The problem with a lot of folks is that when they go to the Fountain of Knowledge, instead of drinking deeply, they just gargle." The truth of the matter is that we know so much less than could be known. And, yes, we're talking about everyone, including the smartest among us. Knowledge is like the Pacific Ocean, and the brightest among us has consumed just a few hundred gallons. Given this, we all ought to be humbled by our ignorance and commit to becoming learning engines for the rest of our lives.

Add that to the fact that the current healthcare system—its leaders, providers, staff, business models, and belief systems—are increasingly under attack from powerful, competent disruptive forces. Learning as much as one can about the coming threats, as well as about disruptive innovation, is the next step for healthcare leaders, both nonclinical and clinical. Now is the time to begin, and there are many opportunities.

The fact that you're reading this book demonstrates that you're interested in learning, whether you work in healthcare or are impacted by the industry as a customer. Everyone needs to be aware of what is beginning to happen in healthcare. We have shared innovation definitions, customer demands, competitive threats, disruptive forces, learning resources, and ideas that should be tested in the healthcare environment.

A section titled For Further Information at the back of this book annotates innovative organizations for you to learn from. We have also included a list of books and articles for those who want to know more. Each will point toward other resources, and soon you will be as immersed in this new and exciting field as we are.

And if all else fails, just Google *disruptive innovation* or *disruptive innovation in healthcare* and countless pages of links to everything associated with the topic will pop up. The content is virtually endless. There is much to learn, and the more you know, the better off you will be. Drink deeply!

Many universities, professional organizations, and similar entities are providing courses on disruptive innovation. There are also large conferences, summits, and executive site visits that are focused exclusively on innovation.

Another idea to foster leadership learning is to visit other organizations—healthcare and nonhealthcare—to see their business models and cultures in action. Alternatively, one consulting firm hosts conferences for innovation executives so they can learn from one another. They offer presentations and facilitate dialogue among executives across the country. It is often the case that visits or presentations like these will help leaders and their teams see a vision they may have not understood before. Or they may conclude that what one organization is doing can't be done at their organization, but some modification of it can. Generally, leaders will return to their organizations with examples to help them understand and explain disruption better; inspiration and energy to get on with transforming their own organization; and roadmaps to follow.

In addition to visiting other businesses, explore entrepreneur or innovation incubators in many cities that are hotbeds of new ideas and models. These are places where cities and universities are collaborating with businesses to develop new approaches to solving problems and to commercialize the benefits of local research and development.

St. Louis has a 200-acre innovation hub and technology district called the CorTex Innovation Community. Cincinnati has a similar area called the Uptown Innovation Corridor. What kind of innovation districts exist in your community? Call them. Book a tour. Go visit. Spend some time there and see what is happening.

A company in Nashville called The Disruption Lab teaches courses and sends out information daily on new, interesting, and exciting innovations of all types and in all industries. Further, they have guest speakers on a monthly basis and host tours to other cities (and even other countries) to explore the latest innovations.

One of their recent trips was to Helsinki, Finland, and Tallinn, Estonia. Terry was able to make this trip and was amazed at what other countries are doing. Some seemed to be way ahead of the United States in transforming not only their industries but also their cities. There are many exciting innovations going on all over the world, and we do ourselves a disservice to not explore what is happening on a global scale.

Build a Culture of Innovation

After the leaders of an organization have engaged in sufficient learning, it is time to begin developing a culture of innovation, or at least greatly expand on the one that already exists. The challenge is to move healthcare organizations away from top-down, authoritarian, spend all day in meetings, passive, and status quo management styles to something that is more dynamic, innovative, collaborative, inspiring, and led by relentless but humble servant leaders.

An excellent book that addresses the type of leadership needed in the twenty-first century was cowritten by Aaron and is titled *Leading Healthcare Improvement: A Personal and Organizational Journey.* Although written for healthcare leaders, it is an excellent transformational guide for leaders in any industry.

> **Healthcare leaders must develop a culture that is constantly questioning, learning, coming up with theories, and testing them.**

Healthcare leaders must develop a culture that is constantly questioning, learning, coming up with theories, and testing them. Think of it as turning all medical providers and nonclinical employees into an army of innovative problem solvers. Amazon is testing hundreds of ideas all the time. When improvement teams come together at Google, participants are given a short period of time (minutes) to brainstorm ideas that will improve a process or product tenfold, not just the 10 percent often asked for in healthcare improvement teams.

And they test the ideas immediately (like next Tuesday) when possible, or in some cases, this afternoon; the sooner the better.

Let us share the relevant practices that drive a culture of innovation and are deemed most responsible for Amazon's meteoric rise from a Seattle garage in 1994 to one of the largest and wealthiest companies in the world:

» **Innovation is driven from the top.** Surveys show that 79 percent of senior leaders across the US consider innovation as one of their top three priorities. Yet the reality is that most of their day is consumed with maintaining the status quo. Amazon CEO Jeff Bezos spends most of his time examining how the world will look three, five, and ten years out. He is focused on results for the third quarter two years from now. He sees his job as identifying and defining the innovation roadmap that will take the company from where it is today to where he wants it to be in the future, on time and on schedule.

» **Ideas are assets.** Unlike most companies, Amazon places an asset value on ideas. Bezos is the Ideator in Chief. He loves unconventional concepts, new technologies, and better ways of operating. He is quoted as saying; "I could fill this whiteboard in an hour with 100 ideas." He believes his function is to create a culture that expects and respects ideas at all levels and acts with a sense of urgency to speed their implementation. His role is to channel this opportunity mindset to every individual, department, business unit, and outpost. He is constantly reminding his people to think longer term, obsess over the customer, and be willing to invent. He wants to retain his emphasis on "Day 1 Thinking"— full throttle attack mode of the start-up Amazon once was. When asked what "Day 2 Thinking" looks like, he answers, "Static, followed by irrelevance, followed by excruciating decline and death." Think of Sears, or some of the hospitals that have already gone bankrupt and closed their doors.

» **Move first, experiment constantly, and fail fast.** With zero background in hardware, and against the advice of everyone, Amazon entered the electronic device world with its Kindle E-reader in 2007. And in spite of numerous setbacks and hurdles, it prevailed and became a game changer. The company realized it could learn new skills if it was willing to assault assumptions. It went on to pioneer the smart speaker category with Echo and Alexa, which now have thousands of things they can do and the list is still growing. Amazon values experiments, lots of experiments. Amazon is willing to move first, to test, and to fail, transforming it into not just an online retailer but a movie studio, a hardware company, a grocer, a web services provider, and above all, an idea factory. The company will often invent something or develop some new capability for its own needs only to find that it can monetize that invention for others.

» **Practice data-driven, customer-led innovation.** Amazon pioneers new approaches to the process of innovation itself. Who thinks like that? One example is data-driven, customer-led innovation. Unlike Steve Jobs who said, "It's not our customers' job to tell what they want next—that's our job," Amazon believes they can listen to customers through the data. They believe that if you're simulating and building models and milking the data, customers will lead them to great offerings. Amazon lets customers steer them and then tries to invent products and services they will love.

» **Promote a clear-thinking, risk-taking culture.** Going along to get along is not a virtue in the Amazon culture. Creative tension, rather than laid-back harmoniousness is believed to spur the best thinking. To be clear, you need to be certain about what you are saying because you will receive a barrage of questions. No single manager has the right to kill an idea. The culture is such that hundreds of managers can green light an idea, at least to the next stage. High potential ideas must meet three criteria: original, scalable, and have the potential to produce a significant return on capital. Bezos wants memos explaining high investment initiatives to have topic sentences, verbs, and clear thinking throughout.

Terms such as *relentless, resourceful, fast, inventive,* and *customer-obsessed* have been used to describe the corporate culture at Amazon. A number of healthcare organizations are working hard to transform their cultures to be more like Amazon's, and we have had the privilege of helping many of them make great strides in developing a culture of learning, improvement, and innovation. One excellent example is Denver Health, a safety-net hospital that has more Medicaid patients than any other hospital we know. And they make it work.

Building on the foundation laid by his predecessor, Dr. Art Gonzalez (President and CEO of Denver Health from 2012 to 2017) turbocharged the organization by building an advanced and amazing culture of learning and improvement. In no small part due to his efforts, Denver Health continuously trains employees with instructors that include executives; have leaders who go outside their offices daily to where the work gets done to learn and coach; and have thousands of employees—including physicians—involved daily in improving every aspect of the organization. They have a very active chief operating and acceleration officer who knows how to pull teams together for large-scale, rapid improvements and breakthrough innovations.

Early in Dr. Gonzalez's tenure, Denver Health began budgeting for and conducting an annual *Shark Tank*–style program where employees and physicians are invited to present new and often disruptive business ideas, which are voted on by the participants of the program. The winning ideas are subsequently implemented by the hospital. It is a lot of fun and generates tons of ideas, many of which are implemented, adding new and better ways to provide care for their patients and new ways to generate revenue for the hospital.

Denver Health also hosts day-and-a-half site visits for executive teams of other organizations so they can see what Denver Health is doing and gain new ideas for their own organizations. Dr. Gonzalez has since retired, but the leaders at Denver Health say they would never go back to the old style of top-down managing that unfortunately is still prevalent in far too many healthcare organizations across the country.

Like Denver Health, we think innovators need resolute and sustained commitment from the top. They need a culture of experimentation that embraces risk and encourages "failing forward". Leaders must ensure that anyone who sees a problem can research, prototype, and test a solution.

For the most part, contemporary healthcare cultures are passive in nature. The idea of their aggressively pursuing the marketplace with a service mentality is foreign to many. They have always had a culture of "if you get sick or break something, come to us." They have traditionally built their hospitals and waited for patients to come to them. They rely on an expert model, or as Christensen puts it, the "solution shop" mentality with highly paid workers providing expensive care even when much of this work could be moved to lower levels and done at less-expensive locations.

Cynics have called this type of culture eminence-based medicine instead of evidence-based medicine, where physicians are rarely questioned and are allowed to practice as they see fit. Except for encouraging yearly physicals, healthcare is a sick care model where the customer is expected, as a patient, to be patient in the waiting rooms. And whatever you do as a patient, don't ask too many questions. It might aggravate the providers.

How many other industries discourage two-way dialogue with customers? Also, when was the last time a medical provider asked for your feedback regarding their service? Healthcare does use vendors to collect patient feedback, but this is typically several weeks old and is of little use for day-to-day management. This model can and must be disrupted by existing healthcare organizations before others disrupt it for them.

Healthcare organizations also have a dismal record of sustaining improvement once they've achieved it. Manufacturing companies (who long ago experienced significant upheaval and disruption) will tell the healthcare industry the reason they cannot sustain improvements is that the idea of standard work is either foreign or new to them. Many healthcare organizations who try to implement standard work soon realize theirs is an opt-out culture, where providers and nonclinical staff think standard work is a good idea for everyone else, but because they are so experienced, they don't need it. Hospitals threaten to hold them accountable, but rarely do. The result is significant variation in practice patterns, considerable waste in work processes, and unwarranted harm to patients.

> Healthcare organizations also have a **dismal record** of sustaining improvement once they've achieved it.

The only way best practices and new business models can be implemented and sustained is if there are management systems in place to ensure standard work is written, taught, and followed on a consistent and ongoing basis. If the current culture is not changed, many innovative ideas that are to be implemented inside a hospital or clinic will not be sustained, thereby wasting a lot of time, energy, and goodwill. The healthcare industry has not been under pressure to actually manage like other industries have been forced to. But with value-based care and demands for at-risk contracts, those days will soon be over.

Develop a Structure for Innovation (Organize for Innovation)

Just as with strategy deployment and performance improvement, a structure for innovation is critical. Innovation-related initiatives should be included in the organization's strategic plan. Furthermore, a disruptive innovation steering committee should be set up to guide the effort. This committee should be composed of executives and physicians, with a champion (perhaps a chief innovation officer) who has overall accountability. Prioritization and deployment of innovation initiatives should be done at this level.

After studying customer-inspired needs, conducting in-depth discussions with customers (including individuals, families, and employers), examining the greatest threats from competition, and exploring disruptive ideas that are already being developed, the disruptive innovation steering committee should be given free rein to determine which disruption models will work best for the organization. They should explore internal and external possibilities, pull suggestions from everyone, and push for new ideas to reduce cost dramatically, improve quality, and enhance the patient experience. They may even set aside money to partner with entrepreneurs who are working to disrupt healthcare. Such disruptors can be funded through joint ventures that are mutually beneficial to both parties, or by finding a way to bring them in house.

If we recall the earlier story about Kristi Henderson, the former chief telehealth and innovation officer at the University of Mississippi Medical Center, her creative (and disruptive) use of telehealth produced a win for everyone in Mississippi. She was an incredible champion of disruption. The UMMC story also illustrates how much an out-of-the-box thinker can accomplish when leveraging technology, collaboration, shared space, and moving work to the appropriate skill level. By doing these things together she was able to increase access considerably, maintain quality, and reduce cost.

With a mandate to test many ideas for change and improvement, incubate new start-up businesses, and explore joint ventures and other collaborative initiatives, the disruptive innovation steering committee can charter innovation teams, select executive champions, and provide time, space, and other resources.

Innovation teams should be composed of emerging leaders who are curious and forward-thinking. Once selected, they should be put through intense training on the tools and concepts of all types of innovation. Facilitators should be trained or brought in. Then ample time should be set aside, preferably offsite and out of sight, for intense uninterrupted work.

Charters for such teams might look something like the following:

> » "We want to start small by developing a health plan for our own employees and seeing if we can provide care for them that is less expensive to them, easier to access, and a great patient experience. What would that look like? How can we design care to keep them healthy and out of the hospital, reduce our cost, and maintain quality?" (We recommend starting by disrupting your own organization first. You will learn a lot and subsequently be better equipped to go at risk to provide true healthcare for other customer groups. If you cannot go at risk for your own employees, how will you be able to do it for outside customers?)

» "If a company, union group, or some other consumer coalition in our area said they wanted this organization to go at risk and cover primary care for 25,000 lives at 20 percent less than they are currently paying, what would business models look like that would enable us to respond?"

» "Design a cardiology business that has higher quality at 20 percent less cost and greater patient satisfaction."

» "Create a plan for one or more of our service lines to become certified by the Employers Centers of Excellence Network (ECEN) as a Center of Excellence."

» "Develop a plan using preventive care and health coaching that would allow us to reduce the annual per employee healthcare spend for large employers by 25 percent."

» "Come up with ideas about how we can avoid building a huge parking garage for our staff and make coming to work easier and cheaper for them."

» "Develop models of how we could use ride sharing to reduce our length of stay and reduce ambulance costs."

» "Develop models for how we might use shared space closer to the customer to make our care less expensive and more accessible."

» "Develop ideas for how we could use 3-D printing to reduce our supply costs."

If these charters seem far out, consider that most of them have already happened.

The role of the executive team and executive sponsor should be to protect the teams from the organizational antibodies as well as general negative thinking. Teams need to be to shielded from sentiments like: "Why do we need to do this?" and "We've never done that before;" and "It's not in the budget." Leaders should allay the fear of managers that new designs will cannibalize their departments, soothe concerns from marketing that the disruptive business will damage the brand of the larger organization, and calm staff who say they simply don't have time to worry about it.

Leaders should encourage the innovation teams not to let *the perfect* be the enemy of *the good*. Following the advice of the lean start-up literature, leaders should insist that teams get ideas into practice as soon as possible (see *The Lean Startup* by Eric Ries). Leaders should also be willing to encourage teams to fail (or as we prefer, to learn) quickly. We believe finding something that does not work, or does not work very well, is not a failure, but valuable learning that can propel people to look at products and services differently.

As disruptive innovation teams start to work, they should be encouraged to review the imagine section at the beginning of the book. Consider the "wouldn't it be nice if…" list of what customers ask for as well as what some don't know to ask for. Further, they should look over the many solutions outlined in previous chapters to spark ideas about what might be done in healthcare organizations.

Finally, they need a process to follow and standardized tools to guide their activities. While a variety of processes could be used, we have included a good one next. And while there is no end to the list of tools and concepts a team might use, we will share a few in coming sections that are especially helpful. These tools include design principles and others embedded in the disruptive innovation process.

Employ Disruptive Innovation Design Principles

While all changes do not result in disruptive innovation, all disruptive innovation requires change. The ability to develop, test, and implement changes is essential for anyone or any organization that seeks disruptive innovation.

Several types of change will lead to disruptive innovation, and these are derived from a limited number of design principles—general notions or approaches that have been found to lead to disruptive innovation. Creatively combining these design principles with knowledge about healthcare can help generate ideas for disruptive innovation.

The design principles include the following, and each is explained in more detail next:

» Move work in time to when the customer needs it.

» Move work closer to the customer.

» Move work to the appropriate skill level.

» Use shared space that is already available.

» Make the product/service easy to understand and use.

Move work in time.

This principle is simply about making the product or service available when the customer needs and wants it. Physician offices are open during the same work hours as everyone else, so to see a doctor, patients are required to take time off from work. And given that it usually takes one to two hours to see most physicians, then another hour or two to get their meds, patients often waste at least a half day to get the care they need.

Illness and pain don't wait until Monday at 8:00 a.m. to strike. Emergency department visits are expensive and are often unnecessary if people could contact a physician by phone or Skype 24/7. So the design question is how can service be provided anytime, all the time.

Often someone who is struggling with an issue doesn't need a physician, but a medical coach who could provide information, support, or direction to help. Again, these needs don't always coincide with the eight-to-four, five-days-a-week time frame.

Another example is that many patients cannot be discharged from a hospital before 5:00 p.m. simply because family members or friends cannot take off work to pick them up. This is a major contributor to the length of stay problem, which is very costly to hospitals. So moving transportation work in time might include the hospital paying for an Uber or Lyft ride home whenever it is safe and optimal for both patient and the hospital.

And what about wasted time? According to research by Uber, automobiles are sitting unused over 90 percent of the time. Hospitals spend millions to build parking garages with money that could subsidize employee use of ridesharing apps, enabling employees to reduce the number of cars they have to purchase, fill with gas, maintain, and pay insurance on. Eliminating these costs for employees would be tantamount to a very nice raise.

And what about expensive time? Another example is to provide coaching and primary care to patients so that they never have to spend time in an emergency room or a hospital bed. That is an example of moving time spent upstream to eliminate the need for more expensive downstream time.

Move work closer to the customer.

> This principle is about moving the work to **where** the customer needs it done...

One of the more important characteristics of disruptive innovation is that it increases accessibility to the service or product. This principle is about moving the work to where the customer needs it done, reducing the inconvenience to the customer, and sometimes eliminating the space between supplier and customer altogether.

The ATM is an excellent example of this. No one has to go inside a bank anymore to make a deposit or withdraw money. Your cash is now available 24/7 (moved in time) in airports, malls, convenience stores, restaurants, bars, bowling alleys, and casinos (all closer to the customer). With credit card innovation, there is now very little need for cash or ATMs. And even credit cards are in the process of being rendered obsolete (starting in China) with WeChat's mobile payment service. Disruptive innovation marches on.

WeChat is a Chinese multipurpose messaging, social media, and mobile payment app. It has become one of the world's largest stand-alone mobile apps—with over 1 billion monthly active users and 902 million daily active users—and is known as China's "app for everything" and a "super app" because of its wide range of functions and platforms.

In addition to its Facebook-like social media and social networking services, WeChat's success has been powered by the platform's mobile payment service, WeChat Pay, which assists with every aspect of a user's life—from shopping and hailing taxis, to organizing hospital appointments and ordering food deliveries. The use of mobile payment services is so prevalent in China that the only people using credit cards or paper currency are tourists.

Now expanding beyond China to other countries, WeChat is exporting mobile payment to the world. Its immense scale will ensure WeChat has a dramatic impact on global finance as people replace cash with mobile payments, and as mobile payments supersede traditional credit and debit cards. Because WeChat allows local merchants to receive payments to their account within a shorter time frame and at a lower transaction cost than credit cards, WeChat could potentially usurp business from the major credit card companies like Visa, MasterCard, and American Express.

The brick and mortar retail industry is learning to their detriment that when you move shopping in time and closer to the customer, many customers like it. There are still those who prefer to go shopping so they can touch, feel, and try on merchandise. But even those people don't want to do that when time doesn't permit or when it is otherwise inconvenient. As nearly everyone knows, you can order just about anything online at any time of the day or night. And most online retailers offer a variety of shipping methods so you can receive the merchandise just about whenever you choose to have it delivered. And you never have to leave the comfort of your home or wherever you happen to be.

From the consumers' perspective, it makes perfect sense to move work out of the hospitals into the large clinics/doctors' offices, and from those to smaller clinics that are even closer to the customer, and from there to evisits and even provider visits to patients' homes.

Advances in technology—including telemedicine and bio devices—provide even more reason to move healthcare to the home whenever it is appropriate. Having devices where the patient/customer can monitor the feedback relevant to their medical condition in real time will get them more actively involved in managing their own care. Also, having medical providers and health coaches available 24/7 to respond to questions via phone calls or texting will reduce patients' anxiety about what to do if something happens. It will also reduce unnecessary and expensive visits to emergency departments, urgent care centers, and doctors' offices. And even if a patient does have to come in, the mini clinic in the local retailer is usually closer and easier to access than the doctor's office.

Move work to the appropriate skill level.

This is about making sure everyone is working at the top of their skill level or license to ensure providers don't overcharge customers by having them pay for higher-level skills (along with higher salaries) when lower levels can do the work just as effectively.

With the available technology, many retailers have given customers (at least those who still shop in brick and mortar stores) the option to use self-checkout. Many customers prefer to perform this task themselves, while others don't, but at least consumers have a choice. And it has been made so simple that any customer can perform the task.

In the now distant past, gasoline station attendants would fill up your car for you, wipe your windshields, and check your oil level as well as air filter. Now that work has been moved to the customer, or to a Jiffy Lube–type establishment. In most fast food restaurants the task of bussing tables has been moved to the customer. How did that happen? We're not sure, but we do know more than a few people who feel guilty if they don't clear their own tables. Some of us are still wondering how the fast food industry got us to that point. As was previously mentioned, ATM technology allowed work previously done by tellers to be moved to the customer to perform. And many customers are glad to do it.

Likewise, TurboTax has made it possible for customers to do the work of the CPA, at least for simpler tax returns. LegalZoom has made it possible for consumers to perform some legal work previously handled by attorneys. Your car now helps you drive more safely and soon will be doing the work for you. Robots now do work only humans could do before. You may be wondering if robots are an example of moving work to the appropriate skill level. In many cases, robots with artificial intelligence and machine learning are indeed able to do intellectual tasks much better than humans. For that reason, many believe it is appropriate to move work to that level.

Amazon's Alexa will be increasingly performing tasks in the home for us, which used to go left undone or that we had to handle ourselves. As we alluded to previously, Alexa and similar technologies will increasingly (and sooner than you think) help people with in-home healthcare.

A friend of ours who is the chief medical quality officer at a well-known hospital still sees patients in addition to his other duties. He is a class act, very conservative, and obviously focused on quality and safety. He openly admits that if the payment structure were at risk instead of fee-for-service, he would not perform 60 percent of the procedures he does as he provides care to patients. He says those tasks need to be done, but not by someone at his skill level. Midlevel providers, nurses, and so forth are just as qualified to perform many of these tasks. This is very telling and something all disruptive innovation teams should closely examine going forward.

Obviously new payment structures will be needed to optimize where the work gets done. Integrated delivery networks like Kaiser Permanente, which own the payer mechanism and employ the providers, have a huge advantage here. We believe this model, if adopted, would greatly reduce healthcare costs for the country. It should be remembered, however, that while under the fee-for-service model the temptation is to overutilize and overcharge (estimates of overutilization range from 25 to 40 percent), in the integrated, at-risk models, the temptation is to underutilize. So it is imperative that high standards of quality and safety be measured and maintained. Patients and employers will demand it.

One more example of moving work to the appropriate skill level involves healthcare transportation. Because we have worked at hospitals that owned ambulance services, it is clear to us that many calls for an ambulance don't really need that expensive level of service. Is Uber Medical the answer for this problem? Can similar services also solve the problem of getting patients to and from their medical appointments?

It is estimated that as many as 3.6 million doctor appointments are missed every year due to inadequate transportation. Not only is this potentially harmful to those who are missing their care, but represents tremendous opportunity costs to medical providers as well as society as a whole.

Even though this disruption will be fraught with political, regulatory, and economic obstacles, it is certain that one of the ways disruptors with at-risk contracts will significantly reduce costs is to move work to the appropriate skill level. Primary care physicians will do more of what specialists do now, and midlevel providers will do more of what primary care physicians are currently doing (this is already happening).

> **...one of the ways disruptors with at-risk contracts will significantly reduce costs is to move work to the appropriate skill level.**

Further, health coaches and patient navigators will provide the care and coaching that other higher-skilled providers don't have time to do. This will include preventive care and ongoing support that has been left completely undone before and is intended to keep patients from becoming sick in the first place. Finally, technology-enabled and better-informed patients will care for themselves even more (and better) than ever before.

A formal study of econsultations by PCPs across ten specialty areas, including neurology, rheumatology, dermatology, and nephrology, confirmed that, on average, primary care physicians were able to address problems in those areas for 60 percent of patients.

When Rushika Fernandopulle, CEO and founder of Iora Health, asked the head of endocrinology at a top hospital what percentage of endocrine clinic patients could be managed by primary care physicians with a little expert advice by phone or email, the answer was a surprising 80 percent.

Use shared space.

One particularly interesting design principle is the notion of shared space. The genius of Uber and Airbnb is that the companies own no automobiles or homes. They profit by connecting the owners of those unused spaces with people who would like to rent it for a while. They maintain high quality by getting immediate customer feedback on the drivers and the home space. Perhaps unused space for healthcare is the patient's home—at least for the care that is appropriate for that space.

Churches and schools (especially in the summer) are often empty many hours a week. Hotels often have space they might rent at a much-reduced rate. Libraries often have beautiful places to hold groups and classes, yet are unused much of the time. What could be done with those and many other spaces in communities that are currently being paid for but not used much of the time?

Make the product/service easy to understand and use.

This principle is self-explanatory. Any time steps can be taken out of the process or complexity can be eliminated, the customer is more likely to use the product or service and tell others about it.

Some people never worry about buying razor blades. They receive emails periodically from the Dollar Shave Club asking if they need a shipment. If they click yes, fresh, sharp blades arrive in the mail a couple days later. That business could even be disrupted if a competitor could build a blade that was permanently sharp, never having to be replaced. So disruption is always a threat, even for the disruptors.

Many disruptive companies are making their product easier to understand and use. Alexa tells us the weather forecast any time of the day and is adding information and services all the time (we can ask Alexa to play the "Hebrides Overture" by Mendelssohn or turn off the lights at night and wake us up in the morning).

> Many disruptive companies are making their product **easier to understand** and use.

Amazon Prime makes it easy to reorder something you have purchased before by hitting the dash button. Newer cars make it easy for you to see behind you as you back up in a parking lot and assist you as you drive to make trips safer. Uber made it easier to get a ride by developing an app where you push a button and a car appears. They also made it easier for business travelers by sending a receipt to their email. And so on…

What about healthcare? PillPack is an example of making a product easier to understand and easier to use, while also making the medication administration process safer. Why would one ever go back to waiting in lines at pharmacies once they have used this service? Could hospitals develop an app that enabled patients and family members to custom order the food they wanted, when they wanted it, while in the hospital? Would it make sense to put the admissions process online so patients coming in for elective procedures could go straight to their hospital room upon arrival (like arriving at a hotel with a reservation)? Could someone make just one app that contains all of a patient's healthcare data as opposed to one for each facility they go to? Could labs be done at home prior to an annual physical so the provider could access and review the results with the patient while they are together?

Labs at home are already a reality. EverlyWell, for example, provides everything needed to collect the specimens for up to thirty lab tests and includes prepaid packaging to ship the specimens for processing. They also include an app to help consumers understand the results.

The opportunities to make products and services easier to understand and easier to use are endless.

DISRUPTIVE INNOVATION PROCESSES

It has been said that disruptive innovation happens when innovation, business models, and technology come together in ways that use lower-skilled workers, reduce complexity, reduce cost, and make the product or service available to more customers. We believe a structured, systematic approach, if followed by healthcare design teams, will result in better products and services that customers actually want. In a shorter period of time with less cost, a team can get a new product or service to market by following a proven process and by using effective tools along the way.

What follows is a disruptive innovation process that will serve to guide design teams and provide them the tools to be successful. This was created by The Disruption Lab in Nashville and is composed of six distinct steps: opportunity, job to be done, technology, business model, experiment, execute.

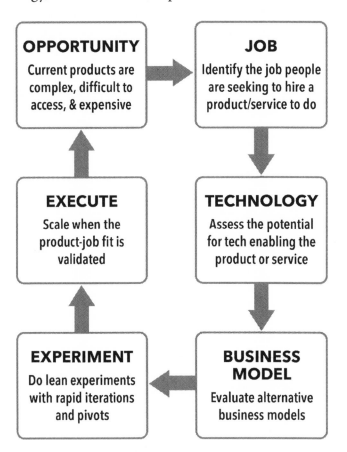

The disruptive innovation process.

Source data for this graphic was used with permission from The Disruption Lab, Nashville.

Process Step #1: Opportunity

Where should innovation teams look for disruptive innovation opportunities? Start with customer experience and identify any products or services that are complex, difficult to access, inconvenient, or expensive.

Since this describes most existing healthcare services, it shouldn't be difficult to find opportunities for disruptive innovation. Teams should ask this question about all of their organization's offerings: "If this was easy for consumers to access and use, what would it look like?" Then generate lists of things that make the targeted products and services difficult to access and use, and then prioritize that list.

> "If this was **easy** for consumers to access and use, what would it look like?"

Visualize a single working mother with three children. One of her daughters wakes up crying with the same earache she had six months ago. The mother is sure she needs the same antibiotic that was prescribed at that time. When Mom calls the doctor's office, they tell her she has to come to the office, the doctor's schedule is full, but that they will work her in. They tell her to come at 2:00 p.m.

She arranges for her mother to take care of this daughter. She drops her other children off at school and goes to work. She gets permission to leave work early from her boss, adjusts her workload with a coworker, doesn't eat lunch, and leaves work at 1:00 p.m. to pick up her sick daughter and head to the doctor's office. Once she arrives at 2:00 p.m. with her daughter, who has been miserable all day, she waits an hour and twenty minutes because they are working her in. Meanwhile, she calls her mom to be at the house when the other children get home from school.

Once they are with the doctor, it takes about two minutes for him to conclude that the child needs (you guessed it) the same antibiotic she was prescribed six months ago. Now Mom and sick daughter face a trip to the pharmacy and a one-hour wait there to pick up the prescription. She calls the dance instructor and cancels on daughter's class that evening, picks up fast food drive-thru for dinner, and gets home with one sick kid to two starving kids waiting with homework, a hamper of laundry, and sixty-two email messages from work.

Do you think all of this would be considered inconvenient by the mom? Unnecessary? Wasteful? On the other side, the doctor's office feels good that they were able to work this mom in on the same day she called. How far would this perception be from what the mother felt relative to the service provided?

Process Step #2: Job to be done

The second process step considers the job the customer needs done. Although it did not originate with him, we were first introduced to this concept by Harvard Business School professor Clayton Christensen, who suggests that we can't reach solutions based solely on assumptions, analysis, or research alone. Christensen argues that we need to understand the individual reasons behind why people do certain things. He suggests that people *hire* products or services to fulfill certain *jobs* the customer needs done. His thought-provoking book on this is entitled *Competing Against Luck*.

Customer surveys and focus groups are helpful but inadequate. To look at a job that the customer needs done requires a much higher degree of specificity about what one is building a product or service (or larger business) to do. The jobs-to-be-done approach considers a far more complex picture, beyond the traditional marketing concept of consumer needs.

For example, when one thinks of people who are obese, what does one think their healthcare needs might be? What progress do they need to make and in what part of their life? What job do they need healthcare to do for them? Do those people need a fifteen-minute office visit and pills to treat the multiplicity of diseases that are emerging from obesity? Or do they need something else? What do they really need healthcare to do for them?

By the same logic, what job does the single mother mentioned earlier need healthcare to do for her? Most of her day was blown. She juggled a sick child, hungry children, and a sick care system, along with her job, dance lessons, and so forth. Her daughter was in pain all day. What are the emotional, financial, and other circumstantial needs she had beyond just getting medication for her daughter? The job this woman needed healthcare to do for her exceeded just getting a prescription.

This way of thinking in healthcare would enable providers to disrupt and think more broadly about what needs to be done to make staying healthy more appealing to consumers as well as to make healthcare itself more pleasant for patients.

In an article in *Inc.* magazine in October 2016, Christensen and his colleagues synthesized *Competing Against Luck* into a series of questions to help innovators design a disruptive new approach (or business) around the concept of jobs to be done. Asking these questions provides a story that may involve feelings, social or familial issues, as well as the more overt practical aspects. This is a different approach to understanding the people healthcare organizations serve and allows them to look more deeply at what should and should not be designed into their products and services.

1. **What progress is the customer trying to make on what problem?** Consider the functional, social, and emotional dimensions of the desired progress. For example, a person with type 2 diabetes might like to make progress on treating her disease, but also on reducing her constant fear of losing her eyesight or having her feet amputated (the conditions of retinopathy or neuropathy). Further, she might want to know if it is possible to eventually get off the medications she is currently taking.

2. **What are the circumstances of the struggle?** Consider the who, when, and where, while doing what of the customer's job to be done. Do diabetic patients even know what questions to ask when they are in the doctor's office? Do they have friends or a support group to talk with about their condition? Are they too embarrassed to talk about their condition because they are overweight? Do they feel guilty about causing their own problems?

3. **What obstacles are getting in the way of the customer making the progress they want?** Are doctors' recommendations realistic, understandable, and doable? What can be done to help the diabetic patient overcome their midnight cravings? Is the recommended nutritionist convenient to access? Is the information about the condition understandable and relatable to patients? Have we made it easy to incorporate necessary behavior/lifestyle changes into their daily lives?

4. **Are customers making do with imperfect solutions through some kind of compensating behavior?** Are they buying and using a product that imperfectly performs the job? Are they cobbling together a work-around solution involving products or processes? Do diabetic patients have inadequate or conflicting information? Have we as medical providers been crystal clear about diet? Do the recommended foods taste good? How are we helping diabetic patients incorporate necessary dietary changes into their daily lives?

5. **How would customers define what quality means for a better solution, and what tradeoffs are they willing to make?** How would we respond if a diabetic

patient said, "I would really work at this and stay on plan if I just had a coach that I could call or who would check in with me on a regular basis, on my time, when I am not at work"? Do our diabetic patients have access to support people who really know what they are talking about and have a plan that has proven to work if patients do their part? Have we made it easy for patients to do the right thing? Have we helped them get rid of the fear and the guilt? Have we provided patients with an app that helps track pertinent information along with meal plans that work? Have we made the new behaviors/lifestyle fun and engaging? Have we connected patients with each other for mutual support and encouragement?

Note: A company called Virta has designed a process that responds positively to almost everything the diabetic patient has asked for in the previous five points, without the patient ever having to visit a physician's office. They have a track record of getting 80 percent of their type 2 diabetes patients completely off all medications. Their approach is an empirically based ketogenic diet and involves care and advice from physicians, nurses, and health coaches, available on a daily basis. They provide diagnostic strips and an app that monitors keto and glucose levels on a daily basis. Virta also has educational material on diabetes, tasty ketogenic recipes, and an online group of patients with which to collaborate and receive support. [Authors' Note: We are not promoting any medical program nor offering any medical advice. This program is described merely as an example of a disruptive approach.]

Process Step #3: Technology

Next, assess the potential for technology-enabling disruptive products or services. We previously indicated that disruptive innovation involves business model innovation and some sort of value network, but technology can be an enabler. Look at what current technology is available to support the disruption.

The process of 3-D printing enables dentists to make materials in their offices that used to be farmed out. It allows surgeons to examine, handle, and practice on exact replicas of organs prior to surgery. Telemedicine and monitoring devices allow treatment to be moved into the home. Remote surgery, in which surgeons control robots from a different site, allows patients to access some of the best surgeons closer to where they live.

Process Step #4: Business model

Evaluate alternative business models. For example, both Uber and Airbnb used the business model of sharing unused space. In neither case was space purchased, but the business model was to facilitate the connection of people who needed to travel with the unused space in automobiles or to stay in the unused space in homes.

To develop a disruptive business model, we recommend disruption teams use the "Business Model Canvas" developed by Osterwalder and Pigneur and outlined in their book *Business Model Generation: A Handbook for Visionaries, Game Changers, and Challengers.*

This tool is used around the world to help people understand a business model in a clear and structured way. Using it will lead to insights about the customers served, what value propositions are offered through various channels, and how to make money with the new model. The Business Model Canvas gets to the heart of the new proposed business proposition quickly without having to spend twelve to eighteen months developing the traditional pro forma with little, if any, feedback from customers.

The Business Model Canvas is one page and will challenge your disruption team to develop the new business model by examining the following:

» **Customer segments.** For whom are we creating value? Who are our most important customers?

» **Value propositions.** What value do we deliver to the customer? Which one of our customer's problems are we helping to solve? Which customer needs are we satisfying? What bundles of products and services are we offering to each customer segment?

» **Channels.** Through which channels do our customer segments want to be reached? How are we reaching them now? How are our channels integrated? Which ones work best? Which ones are most cost-efficient? How are we integrating them with customer routines?

» **Customer relationships.** What type of relationship does each of our customer segments expect us to establish and maintain with them? Which ones have we established? How costly are they? How are they integrated with the rest of our business model?

» **Revenue streams.** For what value are our customers really willing to pay? For what do they currently pay? How are they currently paying? How would they prefer to pay? How much does each revenue stream contribute to overall revenues?

» **Key resources.** What key resources do our value propositions require? Our distribution channels? Customer relationships? Revenue streams?

» **Key activities.** What key activities do our value propositions require? Our distribution channels? Customer relationships? Revenue streams?

» **Key partnerships.** Who are our key partners? Who are our key suppliers? Which key resources are we acquiring from partners?

» **Cost structure.** What are the most important costs inherent in our business model? Which key resources are most expensive? Which key activities are most expensive?

Process Step #5: Experiment

Conduct experiments with rapid iterations and pivots. As was mentioned before, Amazon is conducting hundreds of experiments all the time. Excellent books to help guide you with this include *The Lean Startup* and *The Startup Way*, both by Ries, and *The Lean Entrepreneur* by Cooper and Vlaskovits. The key at this step is to learn as rapidly as possible with as little investment in resources as possible. Avoid any effort that is unnecessary for learning what customers want.

The concept of the minimally viable product is useful here. The idea is to develop the product or service with the minimum amount of time and cost in order to test and validate it. Here we are trying to find out what parts are loved by the customers, what they don't want, price points, and so forth. Get to market as soon as possible, test your value proposition hypothesis with real customers, and use their feedback to modify or discard the product or service.

Process Step #6: Execute

The final step is to make something happen. When the business model is validated, scale up separately from the parent organization and then at the right time move back to the appropriate place within the organization (maybe that's a service line or department). Sometimes good ideas that have been validated in small tests do not work out when scaled to larger or broader sizes. If this happens, the design team will have to decide how to proceed (abandon the idea, keep it but pivot to another version, or rethink it completely based on guidance from customers).

DEFENSIVE STRATEGIES THAT DON'T WORK

Before concluding this section, we'd like to say a few words about what won't work in the long term. The thoughts and strategies we discuss below are those we've seen tried (often) by healthcare organizations as well as other industries while they were being disrupted, losing market share, or going out of business. These strategies didn't work for anyone, and healthcare organizations should learn from these mistakes.

We say trying to make a dinosaur run faster on less fuel is not possible. This thought is a metaphor for what many in healthcare have been working hard to accomplish, and there is no future in it. We suggest healthcare leaders avoid getting caught in the following traps (some of which were mentioned earlier but are worth repeating):

» Believing that disruption will never happen if we just work harder and faster at what we've been doing.

» Pushing medical providers and staff to the point of burnout. You should be working much smarter, not harder.

» Thinking your loyal customers love you so much they would never switch to a competitor.

» Bringing in more and more expensive technology that is not patient-centered in hopes it will magically transform your business.

» Building new hospitals with nice, new features that look good but don't reduce payer cost. Generally, this will not improve performance in an at-risk environment.

» Pursuing merger and acquisition activity to create a monopoly. This is a short-term defensive strategy that won't work in the at-risk world unless it means you can now provide better care for a lot less and are keeping people healthy and out of the hospitals in the first place. Some larger hospital systems are buying up community hospitals and raising rates, because they can. This is movement in the wrong direction and they won't survive the inevitable competition that is willing to go at risk and will lower costs.

» Pursuing efficiency innovation without disruptive innovation. Strategies such as process improvement, PDCA, Six Sigma, and Lean are great at squeezing out waste in current processes and will still be necessary, but they are insufficient. (And we say this having a collective fifty years working, teaching, and consulting with organizations on how to improve their systems and processes and build better management systems.) As we pointed out earlier, disruptive innovation is distinctly different from efficiency and sustaining innovation and will be necessary for your survival.

» Deciding to seek out and focus only on the higher-margin opportunities. This may seem smart but it's just another short-term defensive strategy that will fail. Remember, this is how the American auto industry lost a disgraceful amount of market share to Toyota, Honda, and others. Beware of focusing just on the high-margin care while ignoring the lower-margin business. Work on both. Consider the commoditized care hospitals are currently charging outrageous prices for to support highly skilled specialists who belong in a hospital. Most of the commoditized care will be provided at much lower costs outside of the hospital. If hospitals cannot compete for these customers, they may decide they have to give up the lower levels of care and focus on becoming well known for treating patients that need highly specialized care. To make that work, they will need to greatly broaden the size of their market to include other states and perhaps even other countries.

CHAPTER TAKEAWAYS

Earlier chapters described *what* was happening in terms of market-changing disruptions as well as *what* should be done in the short term to enable the survival of the industry and ensure it is positioned for the future. This chapter presented our ideas about *how* to disrupt healthcare to bring about meaningful change.

Our focus was on creating a culture of disruption within healthcare organizations. We addressed *how* leaders can adjust their organization and build its capabilities around long-term innovation to remain relevant, stay in business, and thrive into the future.

For existing organizations in any industry, disruptive innovation is particularly hard. But our work across the healthcare industry suggests that established organizations *can* disrupt traditional ways of doing business. We know it is possible, though difficult, and have seen examples where it is happening within healthcare. We examined a few healthcare organizations that are innovating in deliberate, strategic ways and cast our net to other industries to share what we learned from them.

We also explored structures, activities, and tools that might be helpful as we embark on this journey of exploration and discovery. We also discussed the challenges required to create a new healthcare marketplace and ended the chapter by discussing often-used defensive strategies that will not work.

4

From Sick Care to **Healthcare**: Who Gets Harmed, Who Gets Helped, and Who Gets in the Way

WHEN PEOPLE LACK A COMPELLING VISION, THEY ENGAGE IN PETTY BEHAVIOR. ENOUGH OF THAT. ENOUGH WHINING. LET'S DREAM BIG. LET'S THINK BIG. LET'S DO THIS FOR ONE ANOTHER!

What we've covered so far will help healthcare organizations survive. These are the near-term tasks needed to change healthcare's current, unsustainable way of business and to meet the emerging threats. These strategies will help healthcare leaders prepare for what large employers are already asking for and what increasing numbers of employers and consumers will soon be demanding.

This chapter makes suggestions for several longer-term issues we believe the healthcare industry as a whole should confront. Moving these larger issues—eldercare, the food industry, Big Pharma, and personal data—will require the clout of the entire healthcare industry. But moving them will go far to improve people's health as well as reduce the cost of care.

IMPROVING ELDERCARE AND
HUMANIZING END-OF-LIFE CARE

Besides taxes, one thing has remained soberingly true despite the tremendous medical and technological advancements that have been made over the years: No matter how careful we are and how healthful our habits, every one of us will eventually die. This inevitably often clashes with contemporary societal norms and modern healthcare, both of which refuse to accept the fact that old age and death cannot be fixed by modern medicine and that we need to find a better way to deal with both.

Despite what we see and hear in the media, fast deaths are rare. The person who dies peacefully from a catastrophic heart attack while sleeping or sitting at their desk is fortunate in some respects. For most people, death comes after a lengthy struggle with an unstoppable condition—terminal illness, organ failure, dementia, or simply the frailties of old age. But while death may be inevitable for all of us, what is not certain is the timing. So patients, their families, and medical providers wrestle with this uncertainty. Too often they struggle to accept that the fight is unwinnable and fail to recognize when continued life comes at too high a price in suffering.

The first question is why so many people in this country are unprepared for the inevitable physical and mental declines that accompany old age. Granted, death and dying are uncomfortable topics for most people, and many simply don't want to think about it much less discuss it with loved ones. As a result, many people hold onto the idealized notion that physical and mental declines will not happen to them and that they (and their loved ones) will live in good health until suddenly and peacefully passing away sometime in the distant future (which they don't want to think about). Atul Gawande described such a fictional view of agelessness in his book *Being Mortal.*

The second question is why the healthcare system as a whole and medical providers in particular are untrained and uncomfortable talking about death and dying with their patients. It's not like we don't know our population is aging, that everyone is going to die, and that older people are closer to death than younger people. Obviously, doctors and nurses are people too, and many of them feel the same discomfort as nonclinicians in the broader society about death and dying.

Equally clear, medical training is focused on prolonging life by treating and curing disease. Contemporary medical training at all levels (MD, PA, NP, RN, LPN) does not even begin to prepare healthcare providers to deal with, much less have conversations with, patients and families about the end of life.

A final question is why the waning days of people's lives are so often spent in institutions undergoing costly and burdensome treatments that have only a marginal chance of benefit. Many of these treatments impair people's minds, sap their strength, and prolong their suffering. Why do people's final days center around unknown clinical routines that cut them off from the things that truly matter in life (mental awareness, family, etc.)? Such tormenting experiences do little for patients or their family and loved ones.

Patients and their families who simply don't want to give up cause some of this. Everyone has a strong innate desire to survive, and many will to do whatever it takes to keep going. Some of this is caused by selfish behaviors on the part of family members (usually children) who desperately want to keep Mom or Dad alive a bit longer ("Do everything you can, Doctor."), without any consideration for what Mom or Dad want or what's physically and mentally best for them.

Patients and their families are also unrealistic about what is possible. Many believe contemporary medicine has all the answers and that whatever is causing decline can be reversed with some miracle medicine or treatment.

These unrealistic beliefs are reinforced by medical providers (mainly physicians) who themselves may have an unrealistic view of what medicine can accomplish and who are far too willing to try something else rather than to give up in the quest to preserve life and do no harm.

Because physicians often view death and dying as a medical problem rather than a human condition, many are reluctant to tell their patients the truth no matter how grim the outlook is. In his research, Gawande found that many physicians are averse to giving a specific prognosis and will propose treatments they believe are unlikely to work simply to avoid having the difficult death and dying conversation with a patient and family members. After all, it's easier and more comfortable to recommend another medical fix than to talk about death with a dying patient.

Finally, consumers (along with the healthcare industry and medical providers) must confront the brutal reality that the older and more fragile a person happens to be, the worse a hospital is for them. In fact, with hospital errors and medical mistakes ranking as the third leading cause of death in the United States, hospitals are dangerous places for people at any age.

For elderly patients, hospitals present a myriad of risks in addition to mistakes, including too much time in bed, not enough exercise, poor diet, and inadequate pain control. Physicians contribute to this, usually based on concerns for patient safety, by confining patients to their beds, hooking them up with oxygen and IVs, subjecting them to unnecessary procedures, overprescribing medications, and depriving them of sleep by ordering vital signs to be checked at all hours of the night.

Lack of sleep and days in bed can cause lasting damage to anyone, but especially to elderly patients who are more likely to deteriorate physically and mentally, even if they recover from whatever illness or injury brought them to the hospital in the first place.

In fact, research has shown that about one-third of patients over seventy years old and more than half of patients over eighty-five leave the hospital more disabled than when they arrived. As a result, many elderly people are unable to care for themselves after discharge and need assistance with daily activities such as bathing and grooming, dressing and undressing, preparing meals and eating, toileting, or even walking.

With this backdrop as a context, what should medical providers do? How can medical providers disrupt the experience of aging and dying to reduce the suffering inflicted on people? How can they ensure elderly patients receive the basic comforts they need most near the end of their lives? How can they make the experience of dying more humane for patients and their loved ones?

Consider our earlier ideal from the consumers' standpoint as you read this section:

>> Care for the elderly and others nearing the end of their lives is affordable, effective, and humane.

>> Perceptions of aging and end-of-life care have been reframed.

>> The excesses of treatment so pervasive in prior medical practice no longer exist.

>> Palliative care is universally understood and widely used to make end-of-life treatment more compassionate and personal.

>> The care for our country's oldest and sickest patients is loving and dignified. In addition to love, these patients receive companionship and help, making sure they're compliant with provider instructions and advocacy.

Reframe Perceptions of
Aging and End of Life

Aging and dying need to be reframed as natural human conditions, not maladies to be treated and cured. Everyone needs to understand that ending your life in a sterile hospital room sleep deprived, hooked up to a ventilator, being fed through tubes, medicated to the point of oblivion, stripped of privacy and dignity, and being kept alive for a little longer like Darth Vader is a fate even worse than death.

We get it that many people are in denial about dying, especially as it pertains to their loved ones. We understand physicians' reluctance to discuss dying with patients and their families or to throw in the towel when something else can be tried. But we also believe it is up to medical professionals to talk honestly with patients about their prognosis, to stop giving false hope, to talk candidly about the process of dying, and to force patients and their families to face the tough reality of death.

It is also up to medical professionals to end the overtreatment that is pervasive in end-of-life care today. Medical professionals need to (and consumers need them to) acknowledge and discuss with patients that it is possible to have too much of a good thing. More treatment does not always equal better care, and prolonging the dying process is not the same as prolonging life.

"Some families, however, cannot face the reality of the dire situation," said Mayo Clinic's Edward Creagan, MD, a palliative and hospice expert, in his book *Farewell*. "No one wants to make a decision to discontinue heroic measures, and without advance directives for guidance, we in the medical community are obligated to do whatever it takes when a family refuses to accept any decrease in the intensity of care. Tragically, many of these patients languish for days."

He recalled one patient who died on day 202 of her time in the intensive care unit, leaving the devastated family to face the grim reality of the limits of medicine.

The amount of money spent in the final months of a person's life is significant, but evidence is accumulating that the proportion of money spent for end-of-life care is decreasing. Other research has found that physicians provide aggressive life-prolonging treatments for their terminally ill patients, often against many patients' wishes, while acknowledging they would not pursue these same treatments for themselves if they had the same terminal condition. Some say many physicians just don't want anyone dying on their watch.

> **Throwing more medical treatment at very sick people... serves absolutely no purpose.**

Throwing more medical treatment at very sick people who are never going to get well or at patients who are on their way to dying—keeping them and their loved ones in an emotionally and physically charged situation for a longer period—serves absolutely no purpose. We believe the primary focus should be on improving the well-being of those who are terminally ill and dying. We know enough physicians who have seen patients die alone in hospital beds who would never want that for themselves or their loved ones.

How would you rather depart this world: at home in your own bed surrounded by family and friends, or hooked up to a bunch of equipment in a hospital being kept alive artificially for a few extra days?

According to the nonprofit Death with Dignity National Center, death with dignity laws, also known as physician-assisted dying or aid-in-dying laws, stem from the basic concept that it is the terminally ill people who should make their end-of-life decisions and determine how much pain and suffering they choose to endure.

Such statutes have been legalized in seven jurisdictions—California, Colorado, District of Columbia, Hawaii, Oregon, Vermont, and Washington—and are being advanced by grassroots groups and nonprofit organizations in other states. These laws allow mentally competent adults (who reside in those states) who have a terminal illness with a confirmed prognosis of having six or fewer months to live to voluntarily request and receive a prescription medication to hasten their inevitable, imminent death.

By adding a voluntary option to the continuum of end-of-life care, these laws give patients dignity, control, and peace of mind during their final days with family and loved ones. These laws also ensure that patients remain the driving force in end-of-life care discussions.

Focus on Eldercare

Elderly patients have always comprised a sizable portion of hospital inpatients, and they will continue to be a growing cohort for hospitals as the age wave laps upon the shores of the US healthcare system. According to the federal government, patients over sixty-five already make up more than one-third of all discharges because nearly thirteen million seniors are hospitalized each year, and their length of stay is longer than stays for younger patients.

Unfortunately, how hospitals deal with elderly patients is a problem. The unique needs of older patients are not a priority for most hospitals, who are so focused on treating injuries or acute illnesses (such as pneumonia or heart disease) that they often overlook other aspects of caring for elderly patients. Furthermore, hospitals face few consequences if elderly patients become more impaired or less functional during their hospitalization.

Hospitals are penalized with fines by Medicare and other agencies if patients fall, acquire preventable infections, or return to the hospital within thirty days after their discharge. But hospitals aren't held accountable if patients lose their ability to walk or function independently. As a result, most don't measure those things. Safety is easy to measure, while quality of life is not. So most facilities consequently value safety over autonomy. But what do the elderly value? (Answer: autonomy.)

Elderly patients are significantly different than their younger counterparts, particularly the very old and the frail elderly who have a higher risk of functional decline as well as complications arising from the treatments they receive. Other challenges in caring for elderly patients include safely dosing medications, preventing delirium and accidental falls, and providing adequate pain control. Because of the unique needs of these patients, some hospitals have begun treating their elderly patients in separate, geriatric-focused units.

The University Hospitals of Cleveland and San Francisco General are such hospitals. Known as Acute Care for Elders (ACE), these programs have special accommodations for older patients and use a multidisciplinary team approach to address their unique needs. Four key components of the program include

» A specially designed hospital environment with carpeted floors, raised toilet seats, and a parlor for dining and visiting between patients and family members,

» Patient-centered care designed to promote independent functioning,

» Early discharge planning, with the goal of returning the patient to his or her home, and

» Regular reviews of medical care to reduce avoidable complications resulting from hospitalization.

Healthcare providers in these settings focus less on the original diagnosis and more on how to get older patients back home, living as independently as possible by minimizing bed rest, encouraging patients to walk around, and helping patients practice doing activities for themselves as much as possible throughout their stay.

Elderly focused medical units are relatively rare—with an estimated two hundred around the country—and even where they exist, space constraints limit the proportion of elderly who can be treated in them. However, such units have been shown to reduce physical and mental setbacks as well as decrease lengths of stay for older patients while allowing them to maintain functional status.

ACE units also showed improved process-of-care measures—such as the use of nursing care plans, physical therapy consultations, and lack of restraints—and improved satisfaction on the part of patients, families, doctors, and nurses without increasing costs. Elderly focused units have also reduced the number of older patients discharged to nursing homes, and one study found they saved around $1,000 per patient visit. Improving treatment and care for the growing elderly population not only benefits older people but also saves money.

Other providers have wisely started programs where they proactively go into patients' homes and assess safety to prevent falls and other potential problems. It is much less expensive to install railings, floor mats, and walk-in tubs than to treat these folks in the hospital after they have broken bones or otherwise harmed themselves. Again, healthcare first, not just sick care.

Make Palliative Care and End-of-Life Consultation a Priority

In the early part of the twentieth century most people died in their homes, surrounded by family and friends. But as time passed, dying and death became medicalized and institutionalized.

Today many people spend their final days in hospitals, nursing homes, or hospice facilities. This is fine for addressing the physical and medical conditions of aging as well as for people who cannot be cared for at home, but less helpful in managing the emotional and social needs of patients and their families, or addressing their spiritual and practical concerns.

Palliative care—specialized care for people at any age with serious illness at any stage—is a response to these unmet needs. The goal of palliative care is addressing the patient's underlying condition, relieving their symptoms, and helping patients and their families cope with the accompanying emotional, spiritual, and social challenges. Palliative care can reduce the stress on patients and their families as well as help them navigate often difficult decisions: How likely is it that the patient will get better? Are further treatments available? Are they appropriate? What does the patient want to happen? Has there been any end-of-life planning?

Palliative care is not limited to end-of-life care but will necessarily play a prominent role in the care of America's aging population. Palliative care will ensure that end-of-life care is coordinated across all medical services, focused on the needs and wishes of the dying person, and delivered by competent, specially trained staff in the setting chosen by the patient (where possible). Such care has been shown to improve the quality of life (and death) and satisfaction for both patients and their families. It can also be provided at no additional cost, and often with significant savings.

The Center to Advance Palliative Care (CAPC) is a national organization dedicated to increasing the availability of quality palliative care services for people living with serious illness. CAPC carries out its vision—palliative care everywhere—in three ways:

1. Improving the knowledge and skills of all clinicians who serve seriously ill patients and their families

2. Helping health organizations to support and deliver high-quality palliative care to patients and families in need

3. Increasing public understanding of palliative care so that all patients and families will know to ask for it when faced with a serious illness

Established in 1999, CAPC led the development of standards for palliative care programs by providing technical assistance to developing palliative care, allowing individual clinicians and institutions to adopt, adapt, and operationalize findings and measures from research settings to the real world of clinical practice. Since 2006, CAPC has been supported by a consortium of foundations and individual philanthropists, allowing CAPC to grow into a leading resource for palliative care.

In 2015, CAPC transitioned to a membership organization in order to achieve the scale needed to increase demand and to support expanding palliative care across the spectrum of care delivery. Over 1,300 individual healthcare entities have subscribed to CAPC's membership model. This continues the expansion of efforts to increase the availability of palliative care services throughout the nation.

There will never be enough palliative care providers in the US, including doctors, nurses, pharmacists, and social workers. Palliative care is a medical specialty, and practitioners can become board certified. Our broader society will need every care specialty regardless of their professional level to have these skills. Palliative care needs to be incorporated into training programs as a requirement for all medical providers, and all should have the opportunity to put into practice what they learn.

Physicians, pharmacists, nurses, social workers, and other healthcare providers should be empowered to advocate to patients for palliative care and to make sure determining what patients value is factored into the best care that can possibly be provided to them. Communication, planning, and involving the family in the difficult and painful conversations people naturally shy away from are very important. All it takes to start that conversation is to say, "I think you may benefit from palliative care, here is what it is, and here are some of the benefits."

Support Family Caregivers

Care options for many Americans are constrained by cost. Fewer than 8 percent of Americans have long-term care insurance, and very few have the personal financial resources needed to maintain care indefinitely in an assisted living facility or nursing home. In addition, public resources are not sufficient to meet the growing need for or expense of care, and even those limited resources are at risk given the country's financial constraints.

These factors—along with research that has consistently shown most people would prefer to receive end-of-life care at home, among familiar faces and surroundings—account for why family members often decide to care for a loved one at home.

Family caregivers' jobs can include medical and nursing tasks such as managing and administering medications, and even providing intravenous fluids and injections. They may also include helping their loved one with activities of daily living such as personal hygiene, dressing, cooking, feeding, toileting, and cleaning. Family caregivers often provide transportation for their loved one to medical appointments, the pharmacy, grocery store, and social activities.

In addition, family caregivers have to grapple with complicated insurance issues as well as legal and financial responsibilities. They are often the primary advocate for the dignity and safety of their loved one, on top of managing and coordinating across multiple healthcare providers. And doing all of this while coordinating with siblings, parents, or other family members makes it even more daunting.

It's hard to imagine anyone who has the requisite medical, business, social work, and legal skills to perform all of these duties. To say it is difficult to function under emotionally charged circumstances, especially with the pressure of a family member's well-being dependent on the caregiver's effectiveness, is a gross understatement.

With nearly 35 million Americans currently serving in the role of family caregiver, there is no question these people augment our health and long-term care systems. The value of the care they provide is significant and would be impossible to replace through increased spending on government programs like Medicare and Medicaid. Yet, family caregivers receive very little support or recognition for their efforts. This needs to change. And nobody is in a better position to help prepare family members to care for our growing elderly population than the healthcare industry.

> ...nearly **35 million** Americans currently [serve] in the role of family caregiver...

So, what can healthcare leaders do to help family caregivers succeed in providing care and meeting the complexity of needs that often accompany old age and disability? First and foremost, family caregivers need to know more about the diseases and afflictions their loved ones are experiencing. An elderly parent suffering from dementia will need different assistance and support than someone with heart disease or diabetes, or who is just experiencing age-related issues.

Medical providers across the spectrum of care (acute-care hospitals, ambulatory clinics, physicians, PAs, NPs, nurses, social workers) should collaborate with each other as well as with medical associations (such as the American Cancer Society, Alzheimer's Association, and others) to provide basic information to family caregivers about the loved one's condition, the normal progression/trajectory of it, and ways to support their loved one.

Family caregivers also need basic instruction on pertinent nursing/medical tasks they will likely perform for their loved ones based on their condition. These may include counting pills, administering medications, and calibrating medical equipment. Family caregivers also need to know what support services are available, how to reach them, and how to partner with health-care and social service teams such as visiting nurses and home healthcare suppliers.

Beyond the medically related tasks family caregivers need to know, they benefit from meeting and networking with others who are struggling with similar experiences. Medical providers can facilitate support groups, or at least help connect family caregivers to existing support groups in their communities.

Support groups serve many purposes, including helping people realize they are not alone, providing opportunities for people to express themselves, delivering information and learn-ing, and affording the opportunity to help one another. Support groups may even motivate friends and other family members to increase their own level of assistance in providing care. Being part of a support group often reduces anxiety, calms fears, and makes participants feel less isolated.

Finally, some caregivers put so much effort and emotional energy into their caregiving duties that they neglect their own well-being. As a result, their own physical, mental, and emotional health suffers. Medical providers can alleviate some of this by referring family caregivers to the appropriate support group. But they can also help by coordinating their healthcare and social service teams to provide the resources, education, and empathy family caregivers need.

Medical providers may also offer respite care services so family caregivers can take breaks to run errands, visit friends, or even take a much-needed vacation. Caregiver stress and burnout are real concerns and should not be ignored. They will not only endanger the health of the caregiver, but also make the care they provide less effective.

Employ Technology to Help the Elderly

We've described how technology can be used to empower consumers with medically related information, to augment the tremendous knowledge and skills of caregivers, and to connect medical providers with their patients. But an impressive array of technology is being developed to meet the needs of a growing elderly population without overburdening the health system.

Such technologies help older people maintain their independence, confidence, and quality of life while enabling them to age in place. Smart technologies using activity sensors, monitoring apps, GPS, voice recognition, and cellular connectivity via mobile phones are creating connected independence that gives family caregivers (who are often adult children, other family members, and even medical providers) insight into their loved one's daily activities and confidence that their health needs are being met.

Other technologies focus on helping seniors maintain their health and wellness, thus preserving their ability to continue living at home. The functions of these gadgets include medication management (for example, providing medical reminders, dispensing medications, tracking medication use), monitoring vital signs, tracking health indicators such as activity versus inactivity, meal planning, encouraging brain games, and providing overall health management support.

Still other technologies help seniors stay connected with family and friends to avoid feeling isolated or depressed. These technologies include simplified computers and tablets, no-contract mobile phones, amplified mobile phones, and video chatting. A final category of health technologies focuses on helping the elderly stay safe at home. These include home monitoring systems and personal emergency response systems that enable anyone to summon help if needed.

AARP provides an excellent summary of some of these technologies to help the elderly on their website (www.aarp.org), as does HomeCare and TheOnlineMom. According to AARP, Medicare and Medicaid may not pay for all of these technologies, but that hasn't stopped the surge of interest in these aging-in-place technologies as more and more people welcome the independence and lifestyle freedoms they provide.

Although older people aren't typically early adopters of new technologies, many are becoming more technology savvy with assistance from others. For our families, helping our elderly parents use new technology has been a wonderful way for grandchildren to help their grandparents with something that is interesting to both generations. And when someone wants to age in place instead of leaving their home, technology can be a lifesaver as well as something that's cool to use.

The big-name tech companies are also getting in on the action to empower older people to live independently. Amazon is developing its AI-assistant Alexa as an in-home health concierge. The inevitable physical and mental deterioration of the aging process is a difficult adjustment. The ability to use their voices to activate assistance and get reminders to stay on track is giving older people more confidence in their ability to live alone and age in place.

An early adopter of Amazon's Alexa and its in-home health concierge is Libertana Home Health, who is using Alexa along with the Amazon Echo to enable seniors to verbally report medical data (such as weight, blood pressure, or blood sugar levels), listen to reminders (to exercise, drink water, eat snacks, take medications), call a medical provider for help, coordinate transportation, and learn about their scheduled social and recreational activities. Not only did all the participants in the pilot program learn how to successfully use and become comfortable with the system, but Alexa ultimately became a companion and friend to the elderly users and helped reduce the loneliness they experienced.

In an even more futuristic vein, the use of digital assistants in the form of robots and chatbots are being explored to help the elderly. Digital companions are being developed to do everything from monitoring chronic health conditions to encouraging patients to stay active and engaged. Digital companions using natural language voice recognition have enabled some health systems to cut back on nurse home visits as well as prevent unnecessary trips to the emergency room.

> Digital companions are being developed to do everything from monitoring chronic health conditions to encouraging patients to **stay active** and engaged.

For example, an eldercare program in Boston called Element Care began using digital avatars on tablets instead of nurses to help selected patients manage their chronic conditions at home. The avatar in the form of an animal reminds patients to take their medications and follow their treatment plans. The avatar can also guide patients through breathing exercises and provide an ear for them to talk to so they don't get lonely.

Indeed, loneliness affects more than one-third of older adults in the US and is a significant predictor of poor health. Elderly people who experience loneliness and social isolation are at increased risk for a variety of ailments, from cardiovascular disease and elevated blood pressure to cognitive deterioration and infection. Helping older people maintain relationships with others as well as remain socially, emotionally, and mentally engaged is becoming an increasingly important role for digital assistants. Avatars on computers and early robots will eventually give way to more cute and cuddly versions that react to sound and touch and mimic the behaviors of live therapy animals.

The Japanese adopted the first generation of lovable elder robots with gusto in the early 2000s, and their softer, fluffier descendants will gain in popularity around the world. Over time they will more closely resemble real animals, and artificial intelligence will enable their functionality to expand so they can help the elderly with everyday tasks in addition to providing companionship and comfort.

Second- and third-generation technology will enable robots to become interconnected with appliances and home automation as well as enable telepresence technology to allow loved ones to check in from afar. Third- and fourth-generation robots will have the ability to take on medical diagnostics and to use facial recognition algorithms to determine how someone is feeling.

Many companies are working to develop more capable and more lifelike robots to help those in need of assistance. The next generations of authentic looking and behaving robots will go a long way in helping the elderly stay mentally, emo-tionally, and socially engaged, as well as feel less isolated and lonely.

But despite all the potential capabilities, robots will never replace real people. There will always be a dichotomy of things robots can do better than humans and things they simply cannot do at all. Older people need long-term supportive rela-tionships as well as help performing the harder and messier tasks associated with eldercare, like getting dressed and using the bathroom. Caregivers will always play a role in eldercare and palliative care and can provide the human touch that no robot will ever be able to.

TAKING ON THE FOOD INDUSTRY

"As grandmothers used to say, 'Better to pay the grocer than the doctor,'" quips Michael Pollan in *Food Rules: An Eater's Manual*. Food and nutrition are indisputably vital for good health and well-being. The food choices we make every day directly affect our health and are part of the foundation upon which a healthy life is built.

Food provides our bodies with the energy, protein, essential fats, vitamins, and minerals to live, grow, and function properly. We need a wide variety of different foods to provide the right amounts of nutrients for good health. Combined with physical activity and not smoking, a good diet can help people reach and maintain a healthy weight, reduce the risk of chronic diseases, and promote overall health.

According to the US Department of Health and Human Services, unhealthy eating habits play a significant role in the obesity epidemic—one-third of adults (33.8%) are obese and nearly 17 percent (or 12.5 million) of children and adolescents aged two through nineteen are obese.

For decades, numerous studies have shown that poor diet (and a few other preventable behaviors such as physical inactivity, tobacco use, and alcohol consumption) poses major health risks that can cause serious illness, even for people who are not overweight. These include type 2 diabetes, cardiovascular disease (which includes heart attack, hypertension/high blood pressure, high cholesterol), stroke, chronic obstructive pulmonary disorder (COPD), osteoporosis, certain types of cancer, and premature death. In fact, these unhealthy behaviors have become the leading cause of disease in the US and a major health concern.

The link between good nutrition, a healthy weight, reduced chronic-disease risk, and overall health is too strong and important to ignore. By making smart food choices, everybody can help protect themselves from these health problems. But it is becoming increasingly clear that the unhealthy choices made by many people are not an accident.

An article in the *Lancet* (a well-respected British medical journal) that examined alcohol consumption concludes that the diseases of unhealthy behaviors are facilitated by unhealthy commercial environments and fueled by corporate interests that place shareholder value above the tragic human consequences that result from them.

Consider the commercial environment in which we live and to which we are constantly exposed. Today's subtle yet always present marketing machine promotes the small daily choices that lead to unhealthy behaviors, which in turn cause disease. Let's face it, "cool" people still smoke and drink in movies; sugar is added to 60 percent of food sold in grocery stores; and the average American spends ten hours a day in front of a screen during which they are inactive.

In addition, corporations make more money from disease-causing choices. Endocrinologist and public health advocate Robert Lustig authored a book called *The Hacking of the American Mind* in which he explains how companies intentionally exploit the neurochemicals and hormones in our brains to make us desire more of their products, which too often contain ingredients that are not healthy for us.

Research has shown that food addiction actually shares common brain activity with drug and alcohol addiction. Lustig's other book, *Fat Chance: Beating the Odds Against Sugar, Processed Food, Obesity, and Disease*, documents the science and politics that have led to the current pandemic of obesity and chronic disease.

> **...food addiction** actually shares common brain activity with drug and alcohol addiction.

If unhealthy choices are not an accident, what can the healthcare industry do to change that? To improve the health of a population through healthy choices, unhealthy behaviors, unhealthy environments, and the corporate interests that promote them must be acknowledged and addressed. Health and health risk mitigation must incorporate healthy daily choices as well as a healthy food environment to promote those choices.

Numerous studies, articles, and documentaries have taken the food industry to task for the unhealthy food they produce as well as the questionable practices they employ to create their tasty but unhealthy foods. We will not repeat any of that, but will instead focus on what the healthcare industry can and should do. And let's keep in mind our ideal future state for consumers with respect to food and nutrition:

» With proper nutrition and increased physical activity, people are healthier and happier.

» Healthy restaurants are among the hottest and most profitable businesses.

» Fast food restaurants have barely survived by introducing more healthy offerings.

» Junk food sales are sinking steadily, and thanks to pressure by health advocacy groups, the food industry has stopped filling everything with sugar, refined carbohydrates, and antibiotics.

» The food industry has also stopped lying to the public about which foods are healthy and which are not.

Pressure Food Producers to Reduce Refined Carbohydrates in Foods

The healthcare industry (including hospitals, healthcare providers, and associations like the AMA) should take on the food industry to force them to quit filling everything with refined carbohydrates.

Refined carbohydrates are also known as simple carbs or processed carbs. Refined carbs have been stripped of almost all fiber, vitamins, minerals, and nutrients that are beneficial for health and, for this reason, are considered to be empty calories. They are also digested quickly, which makes them less filling and satisfying. They have a high glycemic index, which means that they lead to rapid spikes in blood sugar and insulin levels after meals.

Diets high in refined carbs also tend to be low in fiber, and low-fiber diets have been linked with an increased risk of diseases such as heart disease, obesity, type 2 diabetes, colon cancer, and various digestive problems. There are two main types of refined carbs: sugars and refined grains. Unfortunately, these non-nutritious carbs are a large part of the total carbohydrate intake in many countries.

"The food industry profits from providing poor quality foods with poor nutritional value that people eat a lot of," according to Mark Hyman, MD, medical director at Cleveland Clinic's Center for Functional Medicine and the founder of the UltraWellness Center. That's why the food industry should be held responsible for poor diets.

Sugar is a simple carbohydrate that provides calories for our bodies to use as energy. Sugar can be found naturally in a host of different foods, from lactose in milk to fructose in fruit and honey.

There are also added sugars that include refined table sugar (sucrose) as well as concentrated sources like fruit juice, honey, and syrups. It is estimated that the average person in the United States consumes around 19.5 teaspoons, or 82 grams of sugar, per day. That is over double the amount recommended by the American Heart Association, which is 9 teaspoons per day for men and 6 teaspoons for women.

Consuming too much sugar raises the risk of the aforementioned health problems, as well as promotes tooth decay. It is for these reasons that health organizations around the world counsel people to consume less sugar, especially the added sugars.

Sadly, the food industry makes it difficult to judge how much sugar is in the foods we eat. We expect lots of sugar to be present in desserts, ice cream, candy bars, and sugary cereals. But added sugars are hiding in many of our foods, and some have surprisingly high amounts of sugar. Even products that have nutritious-sounding health claims can contain a shocking amount of sugar (you've seen the labels: "added vitamins and minerals," "whole grain," "fortified with antioxidants and fiber," "low calorie," "fat-free," "100% juice" or "25% less sugar").

Further, some brand names or product names sound like they'd be helpful for weight loss (Skinny Cow, Greek Yogurt, Vegetable Chips, Fruit Snacks, Weight Watchers), but even these foods can contain a significant amount of sugar and contribute to obesity.

Refined grains—grains that have had the fibrous and nutritious parts removed—are the second type of refined carbohydrate. Whole grains are very high in dietary fiber, with the bran and germ being the most nutritious parts of whole grains. They contain high amounts of many nutrients, such as fiber, B vitamins, iron, magnesium, phosphorus, manganese, and selenium that are beneficial for health. However, during the refining process, the bran and germ are removed, which leaves almost no fiber, vitamins, or minerals in the refined grains. The only thing left is rapidly digested starch with small amounts of protein that is neither nutritious nor satisfying.

An acquaintance visited a friend in a hospital and said they were serving white bread, potatoes, brownies, and other unhealthy foods to patients. Maybe hospitals should start with their own dietary departments and critically examine the foods they serve patients as well as what they make available in their cafeterias.

We're not complete killjoys and realize that an occasional sweet is fine, but consider Winona Health in Winona, MN. Realizing they needed to be the model of healthy eating for the community they serve, they completely removed sugary foods and drinks from their campus. We're not exaggerating—no more bakery, sugary sodas, candy bars, cookies. Gone! Winona Health took their healthy eating campaign further by reaching out to community organizations to encourage them to do the same when hosting events where food was to be served.

While many people are aware of the dangers of overconsuming foods high in refined carbohydrates, healthy eating is not easy. Our modern food industry is not geared to meeting current guidelines for good health, or for protecting citizens against diseases. Our current food environment undermines healthy eating by pushing energy-dense, nutrient-poor foods that are cheap to buy, heavily promoted, and very tasty. As Dr. Hyman said, "In the twenty-first century our taste buds, our brain chemistry, our biochemistry, our hormones, and our kitchens have been hijacked by the food industry."

The food industry's business model depends on overconsumption of highly processed foods and is fundamentally at odds with people's health and well-being. Here is what the healthcare industry should do:

» Stop letting the food industry determine what food is healthy or unhealthy. The AMA and AHA should create an operational definition of healthy food that includes measures like the ratio of calories to nutrition, the amount of processing that a particular food undergoes, and the presence of unrefined whole grains—not currently on nutrition labels.

» They should then issue their own guidelines regarding what is healthy.

» They should also create a new food pyramid (or circle or whatever shape best illustrates the foods we should be consuming) based on what is medically and scientifically valid rather than what the food industry and agricultural lobbyists pressure the government to include.

» For the operational definition of unhealthy foods, a limit should be set for the amount of refined carbohydrates, sugars, and other nutrients—beyond which a food is deemed unhealthy. For example, any food where the main ingredients are sugar, corn syrup, or concentrated fruit juice would be deemed not healthy. Or any food with more than x grams of sugar would be deemed unhealthy.

» Educate consumers about the mesolimbic dopamine system in our brains that acts as a reward system and help everyone understand that sweet foods activate this system in the same manner that drugs such as nicotine, amphetamines, and cocaine do.

» Create plans to help people gradually reduce refined carbohydrates from their diets.

» Create consumer-marketing campaigns that counter the food industry claims that the global obesity crisis results primarily from lack of exercise rather than poor diet.

» Hold health fairs at local grocery and retail stores to educate consumers about the virtues of eating fresh fruits and vegetables and to illustrate how unhealthy other foods are.

» Gamify health and good eating habits by creating points and reward systems to encourage and reinforce healthy eating and healthy behaviors.

» Partner with local, state, and federal governments to restrict all unhealthy food marketing on television and social media, especially where and when large numbers of children are likely to be watching.

Pressure Food Producers to Curtail Antibiotic Use in Animals

Studies dating back to the 1960s have repeatedly shown how antibiotic use in food-animal production contributes to the growing crisis of antibiotic-resistant infections in people. Calculations using data from the CDC show that about 20 percent of people sickened by an antibiotic-resistant bug pick it up from their food, not in the hospital or from another person.

By now most people are aware that antibiotic overuse in meat and poultry production has given rise to dangerous bacteria that lead to antibiotic-resistant infections in people. *Consumer Reports* reveals that nowhere are antibiotic drugs more inappropriately used than in the meat and poultry industries, where approximately 80 percent of the antibiotics sold in the US are given to animals (including hogs, cattle, chickens, and turkeys) raised for food.

The most recent data from the Food and Drug Administration show that nearly 31 million pounds of antibiotics were sold for use in food animals in the US in 2016. Such overuse has allowed bacteria to evolve so that antibiotics are losing their lifesaving effectiveness for people. According to the CDC, at least 2 million Americans acquire an antibiotic-resistant infection annually, and 23,000 die from such infections every year.

We appreciate the challenges food producers face in keeping their livestock healthy and acknowledge the role antibiotics can play in helping with that. But the levels of antibiotic use in food production far exceed that which is healthy for the animals as well as for the people consuming them and has indeed created bacteria that are outliving the drugs used to treat them.

To counter the food and drug industries' influence on food production will require the collaboration of every professional association within the healthcare industry, along with medical providers. This includes the American Medical Association, American Hospital Association, American Dental Association, American Public Health Association, Infectious Diseases Society of America, as well as the American Academy of (insert names of all medical specialties), and others.

We believe the various medical associations are highly regarded and carry significant weight with the American public. We also believe these organizations need to be more vocal about eliminating the use of antibiotics in farm production. It is, after all, the medical field that is dealing with the consequences of antibiotic overuse and the superbugs that are resistant to conventional treatments.

Their efforts should be joined together as one to push for the adoption of animal production practices that significantly increase the amount of meat and poultry from animals raised without antibiotics and an overall reduction in the use of all classes of medically important antibiotics in food-producing animals, including complete restriction of these antibiotics for growth promotion and disease prevention without diagnosis.

Pressure the Government to End Food Stamp Subsidies for Unhealthy Foods

The food stamp program started off as a well-intentioned way to help people in need by supplementing their food budget. The safety net program has expanded considerably since its humble beginnings and now covers over 42 million Americans at a cost to taxpayers of just over $68 billion annually.

An op-ed titled "Food Stamps Shouldn't Pay for Junk" describes the benefits and downsides of the program, which is officially known as the Supplemental Nutrition Assistance Program (SNAP). The author begins by saying he grew up in a family that used food stamps, but goes on to criticize its current configuration, saying it should stop covering junk food.

The article cites an October 2017 study in the *American Journal of Preventive Medicine*, which found that SNAP participants have worse diets than nonparticipants. This is backed up by USDA data, which show that SNAP participants were more likely to exceed recommended sodium intake levels, receive a larger share of their energy from empty calories, and are more obese than people at the same income level who don't participate in the program.

The op-ed also cites data from the CDC indicating "poor people are 70% likelier to develop diabetes—a disease that puts them at risk for heart problems, blindness, and early death."

The author concludes, "Large industrial food producers love a program that obliges the government to pay for anything and everything they produce. Selling soda, candy, and heavily processed meats is easy when the government picks up the tab. Under SNAP, the big food conglomerates go to the bank while the poor end up in the emergency room." A better approach, he reasons, is to focus the program on affordable, healthy, and widely available foods such as beans, vegetables, fruits, and whole grains.

> **The...healthcare industry should lobby the government to reform the food stamp program to encourage healthier food choices.**

Nobody wants to turn a blind eye toward those in need, but the SNAP program needs an overhaul. The AMA and broader healthcare industry should lobby the government to reform the food stamp program to encourage healthier food choices. Not only will this save money, it will help to reduce obesity and type 2 diabetes as well as lower healthcare costs. As far as we're concerned, this is a win-win for everyone.

Work to Prevent Food Insecurity

The USDA defines food insecurity as limited or uncertain availability of nutritionally adequate and safe foods or limited or uncertain ability to acquire acceptable foods in socially acceptable ways. In contrast, food security is consistent access to enough food for an active, healthy life. In the US, 11.8 percent (15 million) of households were food insecure at some time during 2017. Although this is down from 12.3 percent in 2016, there are still over 40 million people in America living in food-insecure households, including 6.5 million children.

Food insecurity is a complex problem that is closely related to poverty. Multiple, overlapping issues, like affordable housing, social isolation, health problems, medical costs, as well as unemployment or underemployment affect low-income families. Many poor households do not have what they need to meet basic needs, thus increasing their risk of food insecurity.

A *Hunger in America* 2014 survey found that many households served by the Feeding America network of food banks include people coping with a chronic disease that is impacted by dietary intake. In fact, 58 percent of households have at least one member with high blood pressure and 33 percent have at least one member with diabetes. This contributes to a vicious cycle where poor nutrition contributes to worsening health, the expenses associated with poorer health depletes the family budget, which leaves even less time and money to purchase and consume nutritious foods.

The stress caused by food insecurity can be debilitating. When people do not know where their next meal is going to come from, finding food takes priority over things that are less immediately urgent but still important for health (such as keeping medical appointments, filling prescriptions, and having preventive screenings such as mammograms). As Karen Teitelbaum, CEO of Chicago-based Sinai Health System, observed, "Nobody goes in for their mammogram if they don't know where their next meal is."

Food insecurity impacts every community in the United States and includes all demographic groups: seniors, children, rural, urban. Effectively addressing food insecurity requires tackling multiple overlapping challenges with cooperation across all sectors—government, nongovernmental organizations, businesses, and private-sector stakeholders. The healthcare industry can do several things to ameliorate food insecurity:

» Partner with charitable organizations such as food banks, food pantries, soup kitchens, and feeding programs to address food insecurity in the community. One such nongovernmental organization is Feeding America, the nation's largest domestic hunger-relief organization. They work through a network of 200 food banks and 60,000 food pantries and meal programs.

» Work with charitable organizations in your community to expand hunger-relief efforts to promote health and wellness by including health-focused initiatives, targeted programming, nutrition education, and community change.

» Work with charitable organizations in your community to access government funds from the USDA's National Institute of Food and Agriculture programs to support food and nutrition assistance programs that provide low-income households with access to food, a healthful diet, and nutrition education. Three such programs are the Food Insecurity Nutrition Incentive, Community Food Projects, and the Expanded Food and Nutrition Education Program.

» Reduce food waste. The Food and Agriculture Organization of the United Nations estimates that one-third of the worldwide food produced each year (approximately 1.3 billion tons) is wasted or lost. All of this lost or wasted food could feed more than twice the nearly 800 million people who are food insecure. Healthcare organizations can work with local charities to distribute unused and surplus food (food that is still good but past its expiration date) to the needy.

» Encourage careers in agriculture as a health imperative. Global food demand is predicted to grow, so nurturing young people's interest in agriculture is important in creating an effective, efficient, and sustainable food production system to safeguard our long-term food security. We not only need farmers, but also researchers, scientists, and other talented people to merge research, technology, and knowledge to ensure food and nutritional security.

TAKING ON BIG PHARMA

In 2015, American consumers paid over $457 billion for prescription drugs (just over 15% of total healthcare spending), with 6.7 percent annual price increases anticipated through 2025. The high cost of prescription drugs is the result of the increasing number of prescriptions written as well as the high cost of the drugs themselves.

Much of the latter can be attributed to specialty drugs—highly complex and higher-touch formulations that treat smaller cohorts of patients yet have the potential to treat life-threatening diseases. These are expensive to develop and bring to market, and thus command higher prices. For example, Sovaldi, a breakthrough cure for hepatitis C, is priced at $1,000 a pill (totaling $84,000 for a twelve-week treatment). Another is Luxturna, a gene therapy that partially cures pediatric blindness, which costs $425,000 per eye.

Increasing retail prices for generic drugs are also contributing to the growth in consumer pharmaceutical spending. In fact, the cost increases for many generic medications don't seem to be tethered to any form of reality, logic, or morality.

Although relatively rare, whopping price increases with absolutely no justification have become steady occurrences:

» Consider the recent price hike of Nitrofurantoin, a generic antibiotic used to treat bladder infections. Originally available in 1953, its price was increased 400 percent, from $474.75 to $2,392 in August 2018.

» Or what about the sixty-two-year-old drug Daraprim (the standard of care for treating a life-threatening parasitic infection) whose price rose from $13.50 to $750 per tablet in 2015.

» That same year, the price for Cycloserine (a drug used to treat dangerous multidrug-resistant tuberculosis) was increased from $500 to $10,800 for thirty pills.

» Doxycycline, an antibiotic, went from $20 a bottle in October 2013 to $1,849 by April 2014.

» The cost of Isuprel and Nitropress (both heart drugs) were raised by 525 percent and 212 percent respectively in 2013.

» And who isn't familiar with the EpiPen, which was ruthlessly increased in price by more than 400 percent from $50 in 2007 to just over $600 in 2016.

These are just a few of the better-known examples, but prices have increased for hundreds of drugs at rates far exceeding the pace of inflation. Many price increases follow a pattern—a new company (often a private equity firm or start-up) purchases the pharmaceutical and shortly thereafter institutes an astronomical price increase without having done anything to the drug itself.

The result of all of this is that one-quarter of Americans report trouble paying for their prescription drugs. This is significant in that appropriate use of prescription drugs is a powerful way to manage patients' health while restraining costs by helping to avoid costly hospitalizations and other services.

Pharmaceutical companies rationalize the high cost of drugs as essential to funding the research and development of new, innovative treatments. Much has been written about drug R&D as well as the laborious approval process for new medications, and there is no doubt that it is long and expensive (an estimated $2.6 billion in more than ten years, according to one *Wall Street Journal* source). However, we question why US consumers routinely pay two, three, four, and sometimes five times the amount that consumers in other countries pay for the exact same medications.

Consider Nexium, a treatment for heartburn and one of the best-selling drugs in the US. While Americans paid an average of $215 for a Nexium prescription, the cost for Dutch consumers is $23, in England the cost is $42, and in Spain the price is $58. Or take Humira, another popular medication used to treat common conditions like arthritis and psoriasis. The average cost of a Humira prescription in the US is $2,669, compared to $1,362 in England and $822 in Switzerland.

The same pattern holds true for many other medications. A leukemia drug called Gleevec is significantly more expensive in the US ($6,214) compared to anywhere else (Switzerland = $3,633, Canada = $1,141, New Zealand = $989). And American consumers pay four times as much for multiple sclerosis drug Copaxone ($3,903) as those in New Zealand ($898) or England ($862). The list of examples is seemingly endless.

Do you remember Sovaldi, the breakthrough cure for hepatitis C we mentioned at the beginning of this section? Although the cost for this drug regimen in the US is $84,000 ($1,000 per pill), generic equivalents sell for around $4 per pill in India.

There is nothing different about any of the aforementioned drugs from one country to the next—they are identical. The difference is that American consumers are caught between a distorted market in this country and the single-payer systems in other countries that dictate the prices they are willing to pay for medications.

One reason our drug prices are so high is that nearly all countries except the US have policies to lower drug prices, including price controls, regulations that limit the profitability of drugs, reference pricing, and cost-effectiveness thresholds. Countries with single-payer health systems pay less for the drugs they use, but the cost to their citizens is paid in the form of reduced access. For example, cost-effectiveness thresholds used by the National Health Service in the United Kingdom (the country's primary purchaser of drugs) frequently do not cover therapies whose "cost per quality-adjusted life year gained" exceeds $50,000 per year.

> **One reason our drug prices are so high is that nearly all countries except the US have policies to lower drug prices...**

As another example, the number of available medications is typically less in countries with nationalized health systems. For example, of seventy-four cancer drugs launched between 2011 and 2018, 95 percent are available in the US, while only 74 percent were available in the UK. Those percentages drop even further in Japan (49%) and Greece (8%). The bottom line is that countries with single-payer systems save money by denying treatments to their people.

With respect to availability, medications that are approved in single-payer countries are delayed in reaching patients. These countries have drawn-out deliberations regarding how much the health system will pay, which delays the availability of these pharmaceuticals by an average of seventeen months. In contrast, approved drugs are available almost immediately in the United States. Better availability and quality of care is why America outpaces many single-payer countries on cancer survival rates.

In more limited circumstances, some less developed countries go so far as to violate patents and produce their own generic versions of drugs. As a result of all these factors, American consumers end up subsidizing the cost of medications for everyone else.

As if the surreal pricing for medications and the fact that Americans bear the brunt of the financial burden of drug costs for the entire world weren't bad enough, pharmacy benefits management companies are ripping off consumers through various "administrative" fees.

Express Scripts is facing a class-action lawsuit in Pennsylvania for overcharging to provide patient records to patients who request them. This is the third such suit as similar claims have already been made in Kentucky and Florida. What's at issue is the flat fee of $75 to $90 the company charges to fulfill any request for pharmacy records. Many people—including us—feel this is ridiculous.

But why does drug price gouging in the US seem a normal part of the unreality industry of healthcare?

We understand that the pricing of any medication is both science and art and that many different factors must be considered. What is this medication's clinical value? Is it prolonging people's lives? Is it helping patients live better? How does the price compare to medical interventions? How does it compare to other similar drugs? Are there even competing drugs? Will insurers pay for the drug? How much will they pay? What will the average copay end up being? Can consumers afford this level of copay? And the list goes on. The heart of the problem is a payment system that is not consumer-driven or market based.

For newer, branded drugs the existing patent system provides drug manufacturers a monopoly, which they exploit to the fullest. And even when the original patents expire, pharmacy companies go to great lengths using various contrivances to keep prices high. The most common tactic is to obtain patent extensions (and retain monopolistic pricing) by expanding the drug's use with other patient cohorts or even for other conditions. Patent extensions may even be granted for superficial tweaks such as the addition of a timed-release formula or changes to a pill's coating.

From 2005 to 2015, three-quarters of new drug patents were for drugs already on the market, and of the roughly 100 best-selling drugs, more than 70 percent had their patent protection extended at least once, while nearly half were on their third or more patents. Of the twelve best-selling drugs in the US, drug companies filed 125 patents during that period, and 71 were granted.

A well-known example of a patent extension is Lipitor, a drug that fights cholesterol. Several extensions of its patent term, including one for pediatric use, gave Lipitor's manufacturer nearly four additional years of protection from generic competitors. It is estimated that the company took in $24 billion more during this extension period than if the drug had entered the generic category when originally scheduled.

For generic drugs, much of the pricing problem is directly attributable to insufficient competition. Substantial price hikes occur and persist because only one company makes a particular drug, or because manufacturers raise prices in lockstep, which is possible because so few manufacturers compete in many drug categories. Rather than competing for customers by undercutting other makers' prices, when one raises its prices, the others follow. This kind of behavior for drug pricing defies normal market behavior as well as traditional economic theory and signals that something is amiss.

Another factor causing high drug prices in the US is the existence of group purchasing organizations (GPOs) and pharmacy benefit management (PBM) companies.

The first GPO started in New York City in 1910 as a nonprofit coop, where hospitals joined together to purchase supplies in bulk. Like today's Costco or Sam's Club, participating hospitals paid membership dues to be part of the buying coalition and to cover administrative expenses. Other GPOs formed and functioned like this, and the coop model worked well for many decades because they served member hospitals.

But in 1987 GPOs became exempt from laws against taking rebates/kickbacks from suppliers. They soon began charging fees to manufacturers (who paid to gain exclusive access to their members) and began giving members a cut of the GPO's fees. In 2003, pharmacy benefit management (PBM) companies petitioned to be exempted from laws against kickbacks (which Congress approved) and quickly took a prominent role in this misadventure.

GPOs/PBMs use secret contracts to manipulate pricing. Manufacturers and distributors that are unwilling or unable to pay the kickbacks are simply removed from the supply chain. Predictably, this has given rise to a pay-to-play system where suppliers pay fees (often exorbitant) to the GPOs/PBMs in return for contracts giving their products exclusive access to GPO-member hospitals and PBM-preferred distributors.

What is most perverse about these arrangements is that physicians are not the ones who choose which drugs, medical devices, and supplies they use for their patients. Instead, GPO/PBM purchasing agents make those decisions based not on what is best for patients, but on how much kickback revenue these products generate for the GPO/PBM. As a result, patients and medical providers are often denied access to lifesaving, cost-effective goods, and the healthcare system experiences frequent supply disruptions.

> Drug pricing... is driven by a **distorted market** and price opacity.

Drug pricing, therefore, is driven by a distorted market and price opacity. We are firm believers in free and open markets, where consumers are in control and can easily shop around for the healthcare providers as well as medications that deliver the best service and outcomes at the most reasonable prices. But it is clear that drug pricing, like the broader US healthcare system, does not operate like anything resembling a free market.

As we've said before, healthcare is another world. Kabuki drug pricing must be added to the Alice in Medicine Land experience most consumers and patients have with healthcare. The current state of costs and pricing for medicines—like the rest of the healthcare system—is bewildering, irrational, and anything but consumer-driven.

Given the scale of healthcare and the proportion of overall spending devoted to medications, finding ways to reduce prescription drug spending without harming patients and without undermining manufacturers' capacity to innovate and develop new medications is essential. It's easy to see changes to government regulations as the only response to lowering drug prices.

Indeed, a big part of the solution must include changes to various rules and regulations that keep drug prices high. We will address these. But we also focus on the economic lever of price transparency, which has the potential to improve pricing by unleashing the power of competitive forces.

Accelerate the FDA Drug Approval Process

The Food and Drug Administration has already worked to speed up approval for generic drugs, but it must be accelerated even more for both generic and new medications. A faster drug approval process will enable new medications to reach sick patients faster and allow drug producers to begin profiting from their discoveries more quickly.

Several programs to accelerate the FDA's drug approval process have proven successful. A fast-track program initiated in 1997 shaved approximately one year off an average of eight years from the beginning of clinical trials to FDA approval. A second program started in 2012 focused on compressing clinical trials and streamlining the FDA's evaluation process for experimental drugs that could potentially provide breakthrough treatments for diseases.

Half the drug candidates who attained breakthrough approval with an expedited designation took an average of 4.8 years from the beginning of clinical trials to FDA approval, compared to an average of eight years for drug candidates that did not receive the expedited designation. These and other fast-track programs (such as accelerated approval for drugs whose trial results are believed likely to predict clinical benefit) should be validated and expanded.

Liberalize Access to the Generic Drug Market

Many of the pricing problems in the generic drug market are directly attributable to insufficient competition. In December 2013, seven generic equivalents were introduced for the branded antidepressant Cymbalta. Within a month the price dropped 27 percent, and the addition of four more generic equivalents slashed the price in half by the end of 2014.

Although the FDA has the authority to prioritize review of generic drug applications when only one manufacturer is on the market, too few drugs are getting that expedited review. There is a backlog of pending applications from generic drug manufacturers that want to enter the market. Until Congress gives the FDA the resources it needs to process these applications more quickly, the FDA should prioritize applications for generic drugs that have experienced significant price hikes.

Congress should also liberalize access to the US generic drug market by relaxing the FDA's grip on entry. Currently, the FDA alone can approve generic drugs for use in this country. Why not grant reciprocity to any company that qualifies to sell a generic drug in another developed country (such as England, France, and Israel) to sell the same drug in the US without having to go through the FDA approval process? Does anyone think the FDA-equivalent regulatory bodies in those countries would allow unsafe products to reach their consumers?

Reduce Exclusivity Time to Encourage Generic Biologic Drugs

Another solution is to focus on lowering the price of biologic drugs—those deemed by the FDA to be molecularly similar to the branded version. These generic biologic drugs are the fastest growing component of pharmaceutical costs. According to Thomas Burton, reporting in the *Wall Street Journal*, it is estimated that the introduction of biosimilars will cut drug spending by $44.2 billion by 2024. In Europe, biosimilar competitors are typically priced 30 percent below their brand-name equivalents—savings that could be replicated in the US as specialty drugs come off patent.

So why not reduce the length of guaranteed protection of brand-name biologics from generic competition from twelve to eight or six years? Why not do this for all new drugs? This reduction in the exclusivity period would still provide ample time for drug manufacturers to enjoy monopolistic pricing and recover development costs, but would also encourage innovation, increase market competition, and ultimately speed more affordable generics to the market.

Repeal the Safe Harbor Law

The 1987 Medicare Anti-Kickback Safe Harbor law unintentionally created a $600+ billion nationwide distribution monopoly of medical supplies and medications. By legalizing contracts and unsavory practices that would be criminal in any other industry, this misguided statute gave rise to a pay-to-play system that collects fees (including administrative fees, marketing fees, advances, conversion fees, pre-bates, rebates, and sharebacks) simply to allow a given medication or medical device to gain access to the healthcare marketplace. These fees, which artificially inflate the cost of these supplies and medications, add an estimated $200 billion of unnecessary expense to American healthcare every year.

Today, the GPO side of the healthcare industry is highly concentrated, with four supersized GPOs controlling purchasing for 90 percent of the medications and supplies used by medical providers in the United States. In turn, the GPOs rely on an equally concentrated PBM sector where three enormous distributors control over 80 percent of the PBM market and more than 70 percent of all prescriptions dispensed in the US.

As physicians C. L. Gray and Robert Campbell noted, "To give a sense of the magnitude and power of this distribution monopoly, in December of 2017, CVS Caremark (the largest PBM) announced its $69 billion purchase of Aetna (the nation's largest health insurer). This is the market equivalent of a trucking company that delivers soft drinks purchasing Coca-Cola or Pepsi."

On January 31, 2019, the US Department of Health & Human Services issued a proposed rule that would remove the safe harbor for drug rebates. We hope this works its way through Congress and gets passed in a timely manner. Repealing this law would be a giant leap toward creating free and open markets as well as reducing the bewildering, irrational, and anything-but-consumer-driven Kabuki drug pricing that we currently have. It is estimated that it would reduce costs of drugs and healthcare supplies by an estimated 30 percent and save Medicare and Medicaid approximately $75 billion annually. In addition, renewed free-market competition would produce additional innovation and further cost reductions over time.

Allow Medicare to Negotiate Drug Prices

Providing health insurance coverage for 59.1 million Americans over the age of sixty-five, Medicare is the second largest health plan in the US, behind only United Health Group with its 70 million covered lives. In terms of retail pharmaceutical spending, Medicare accounted for 29 percent of total spending in 2016.

Unfortunately for taxpayers and the elderly, current federal law prohibits Medicare from negotiating drug prices with manufacturers or making decisions about which drugs it covers. This insane situation means Medicare must cover FDA-approved drugs regardless of their cost and even if they aren't an improvement over what currently exists. Pharma companies naturally view this as a "sky-is-the-limit" condition regarding pricing for this consumer bloc.

> ...current federal law prohibits Medicare from **negotiating** drug prices with manufacturers...

The situation with Medicare stands in stark contrast to that of Medicaid (where pharma companies are required to provide drug price rebates) and the Veterans Health Administration (where pharma companies cannot charge more than the lowest price paid by any private-sector purchaser). Imagine if the HHS Secretary was not only able to use the clout of Medicare's 59 million beneficiaries to bargain with pharmaceutical companies regarding drug prices, but also to cover fewer medications. The savings would be tremendous.

The VHA is able to purchase drugs that are approximately 40 percent less expensive than what Medicare pays, and it is estimated that allowing Medicare to negotiate prices could produce as much as $16 billion in annual savings for taxpayers, according to a 2015 report by Carleton University in Ottawa, Ontario, and Public Citizen, a public advocacy group. Research by the Henry J. Kaiser Family Foundation found that 92 percent of the American public favors allowing Medicare to negotiate drug prices. So if our government truly represents the people, what's the holdup? This is one of few areas where there is near unanimous agreement across political lines.

Allow US Consumers to Buy Prescription Drugs Anywhere

As we illustrated previously, consumers in the US pay significantly more than people in any other country for the exact same drugs. There is nothing different about any of these pharmaceuticals from one country to the next—they are identical. Under current US law it is illegal to reimport prescription drugs that have been exported to other countries, or to bring in substances that are banned under US law. A number of lawmakers over the years have attempted to change this, and such efforts are receiving renewed attention from the current administration.

To us the solution is very simple—overturn any and all regulations limiting consumers' ability to purchase FDA-approved medications from anywhere in the world. We're not talking about some local brew cooked up by a witch doctor in a remote part of the world. We're talking about medications approved by the FDA and sold around the world at prices that are up to four times less expensive than the exact same drugs in this country.

So why not work to let Medicare, Medicaid, and the VHA get the best price offered anywhere in the world? Why not let private-sector insurance companies and US consumers do the same so they can search for the best deal anywhere in the world? We do it routinely for nearly every other product and service—why not for medications? Such a move promises immediate and significant savings for consumers and fewer headaches for medical providers across the country.

Create Real Transparency for Drug Prices

We've mentioned a few things the government could do to help rein in drug prices, and many of these are necessary to create a free and open consumer-driven market that enables people to easily shop around for the best deal possible. But at the same time, pricing transparency must be created. Most consumers understand there is no formula for pricing new medications and that many factors must be considered.

But what's true for the broader healthcare industry also holds for prescription medications—pharmaceutical pricing is largely unknown by consumers, who are unable to compare prices and shop around for the best deal, and who have virtually no incentive to do so in the first place because insurance companies typically cover drug payments. And good luck if you attempt to price compare.

On several occasions over the years we have contacted different pharmacies to inquire about the cost of particular medications that had been prescribed for us. Every time we were told that a price could not be provided because it depended on our insurance. When informed of our insurance, the pharmacies still couldn't tell us a price because they would have to first process the prescription. Try it yourself and see how much time and effort must be expended to get a price quote for a single medication at one pharmacy.

Improved understanding of how pharmaceutical companies price their products would help consumers determine whether such high costs are justified. And published prices would enable consumers to compare and shop around.

In addition, consumers currently have no way to know whether a newly approved (and more expensive) medicine works better than those already on the market. In theory, drugs that cure diseases would be priced higher than medications that don't improve on existing treatments. Creating a value-based approach to drug pricing—by increasing the availability of comparative research showing the efficacy of drugs treating the same conditions in a manner safe for consumers—would contribute to price competition and reduce spending on unnecessary or ineffective treatments.

Several exciting moves are happening that we believe will transform the overall healthcare system as well as increase the downward pressure on pharmaceutical prices. First and foremost is the emergence of at-risk organizations. The hospitals that are part of the Employers Centers of Excellence Network (ECEN) and Walmart's Centers of Excellence program as well as the health

> Several exciting moves are happening that we believe will **transform** the overall healthcare system...

systems who have contracted directly with large employers such as Boeing, GM, and Disney are all examples of hospitals and health systems taking responsibility for the cost and quality of the care they provide.

Pushed to do so by large employers, these at-risk medical providers will drive fundamental market changes and will incorporate more effective ways to evaluate real-world evidence on the value of the equipment, supplies, and medications they use to treat their covered populations. They will also include risk-based contracts with pharmaceutical companies to mitigate financial exposure, better ways to aggregate purchasing power, and greater transparency regarding drug pricing.

New pathways for drug development are being explored, which promise faster medication development cycles. One is the New Pathways to Drug Discovery (NPDD), which is a multidisciplinary collaboration across the University of Connecticut. Capitalizing on existing intercampus strengths in clinical medicine, drug discovery and development, genomics, molecular biology, and a host of other science disciplines, the mission of the NPDD collaboration is to apply new discoveries in the clinical and basic sciences to the development of therapeutic and diagnostic agents for the treatment of human diseases.

Another route for the future of drug development may be targeting disease pathways rather than single genes and their products. Researchers at several universities and pharmaceutical companies are investigating the complex molecular pathways that control a cell's activities. Although more complicated than it seems, this approach is revealing connections among diseases that seem very different and offers high hope for understanding and addressing different diseases.

A third approach comes from the tech sector, where CRISPR pioneer Feng Zhang has founded a biotech upstart with big plans to speed new drug development. They plan to employ a new CRISPR system with a platform for drug development built around artificial intelligence, genome sequencing, gene synthesis, and screening efforts to find new molecules. Using the new CRISPR system to characterize proteins, the group plans to play a role in the ongoing integration of computational science in drug discovery, by looking to shorten development timelines and improve on some incredibly bad failure rates.

While these and other approaches will reduce the time required for new drug development, the rise of 3-D printing has the potential to fundamentally alter the manufacturing of drugs. Already used to make everything from car parts to toys to blood vessels, 3-D printing may one day enable people to make their own medications at home.

Researchers around the world are working to enable 3-D printers to synthesize pharmaceuticals and other chemicals from simple, widely available starting compounds. By digitizing and hence democratizing chemistry, they believe this will ultimately allow nonspecialists to synthesize almost any compound any-where in the world.

According to one of the researchers, "This approach will allow the on-demand production of chemicals and drugs that are in short supply, hard to make at big facilities, and allow customization to tailor them to the application." Ultimately, this could facilitate the production of medicines used too rarely to justify conventional commercial production, as well as for use in remote settings.

There are many technical and regulatory hurdles to over-come, but we trust science, technology, and the insatiable human spirit will find better, faster, safer, and easier ways, eventually surmounting these obstacles. Competition works elsewhere and it can work in healthcare.

ENSURING PERSONAL DATA SOVEREIGNTY

We produce a prolific amount of information regarding our locations, shopping tendencies, browsing patterns, reading habits, and just about everything we do online is tracked. As more health data move online, our personal health information will constitute an ever-increasing proportion of this data stockpile. But in terms of data and privacy, consumers have lost—or in many instances voluntary surrendered—control over their digital lives.

Consumers are frequently presented with lengthy terms and conditions that offer little choice other than to hand over control of their digital trails. As a result, consumers do not own their data and are not empowered by it. Instead, the companies who control the technologies, platforms, and apps that contain our data wield increasing influence over our everyday lives. They operate in opaque ways and are largely unaccountable for their decisions and actions. Our data have become a valuable resource. But as a currency of the digital world, our data are locked away and exploited by these companies for their own commercial and financial gains.

It's little wonder why patients are always last in line to obtain their own medical data.

Nor are our data secure. In recent years data breaches, flagrant privacy violations, and a cavalier approach to the protection and use of consumer data by some companies have come to light more frequently. The following are just a few of the high-profile breaches most people have heard about—Facebook, Equifax, Anthem, eBay, JP Morgan Chase, Home Depot, Yahoo, LinkedIn, Target, Adobe, US Office of Personnel Management, and the list goes on.

In fact, scores of data breaches happen daily and in too many places to keep count, and most aren't widely publicized. But when they are publicized, it's hard to know what constitutes a truly serious breach. Is it the size of the organization impacted? Is it the size of the breach? Is it the number of records compromised? Or is it the amount of damage the breach caused for consumers, companies, or insurers?

The issues regarding data ownership and security are also true for consumers' health records. Breaches and cyberattacks are ongoing threats in the healthcare industry, and the reality is that patient data and potentially even patient lives are at stake. With increased technology and digital connectivity comes the increased exposure to cyberattacks that can impact patient care delivery, safety, and privacy. Due to the numerous channels through which healthcare data travel, healthcare organizations are particularly vulnerable. The need to protect patient data has never been more critical.

Unfortunately, the IT departments within many healthcare providers are consumed with simply keeping their systems operating at optimum performance. This often ties up most of the IT department's resources. It is difficult for a healthcare IT department to employ the technology and security expertise necessary to develop and maintain an effective security stance. Many also lack the budget and the time required to remain up-to-date on the numerous threats facing their organization. Hence, cybersecurity is an evolving battlefield confronting the healthcare industry.

In addition to the myriad internal challenges confronting healthcare organizations, consumers are becoming increasingly protective of their data as well as of online information about them. The Nashville-based Disruption Lab has identified personal data sovereignty as a megatrend that will impact everyone and have widespread implications, as consumers demand more control over their own data and increased transparency regarding how their data are used. Healthcare companies that fail to address these legitimate concerns will suffer.

Let's recall the ideal scenario we imagined a healthcare system to be as we explore ways the system can be disrupted with respect to our data:

» In terms of data and privacy, consumers have complete control over their digital lives, especially as it pertains to their health and health records.

» No longer are consumers presented with lengthy terms and conditions that give them little choice other than to give up control over their digital footprints.

» No longer are the technologies and platforms that contain consumers' data—and wield increasing influence over their everyday lives—opaque and largely unaccountable.

» No longer are health data locked away and exploited by companies for commercial gains.

» New standards of privacy and control are in place that ensure personal data sovereignty.

Make the EU's General Data Protection Regulation a Standard

The European Union has gotten in front of the data sovereignty megatrend with the implementation of the General Data Protection Regulation (GDPR), which took effect on May 25, 2018. Designed to modernize laws that protect the personal information of individuals, these regulations give European citizens easier access to the data companies hold about them, more control over what data organizations can collect about them, how they collect it, and what it is used for. Citizens can also demand to see what data are held on them and request that their personal data be deleted.

The GDPR also places obligations on organizations that handle data relating to EU citizens, even if they are based outside the EU. These obligations are to protect this information and to be transparent about how it is going to be used. Any organization wanting to do business in the EU will have to comply with the GDPR or face significant fines.

There is absolutely no need for any organization anywhere in the free world to wait any longer. Simply adopt the GDPR and make it your universal standard. Apply it to all of your customers, regardless of where they are located. Don't wait for the US government to pass similar legislation. Take the lead and make GDPR your default for customer data and privacy.

In terms of other ideas, a British-based global innovation foundation called Nesta provides some food for thought. They published a report titled "Me, My Data and I: 9 Projects Helping People Reclaim Control over Their Personal Data," which describes nine disruptors that are helping consumers reclaim control over their personal data.

What follows is a summary of four of the most relevant of these disruptors. Some have created technologies that make new standards of privacy and control possible. Others are digital platforms that help people unlock personal and public benefits with their data, while others are groups and collectives that are raising awareness and enabling people to take action.

Undoubtedly, there are other such disruptors focusing on personal data sovereignty. But these summaries are intended to provide ideas for what the healthcare industry can potentially do now to create the ideal future of a more consumer-centric view of data in healthcare.

MIDATA.coop

MIDATA.coop is a Swiss cooperative that gives people control over their medical data. Users can collect a variety of health-related information, including their hospital records, genetic testing results, data produced by fitness trackers, and other experiential data, and safely encrypt and store it in a local cloud. The user can then track their progress or share the data with whomever they want: their doctor, family members, or medical researchers where their data could prove useful.

MIDATA.coop believes data are best seen as a common resource and encourages users to voluntarily and freely share their data with researchers to help with medical research users feel strongly about. The founders believe consumers/patients gain collective influence by pooling data together, creating a valuable resource that medical researchers can access on certain terms (such as openness about the results of their research).

Though a fairly young initiative (founded in 2015), it has already seen some successes. The first pilot saw post–bariatric surgery patients recording health data like their weight loss and sharing it with doctors investigating the postoperative recovery period. The latest study examined a drug's effect on multiple sclerosis patients by analyzing the data they input about motoric and cognitive capabilities on an app. Since late 2017 anyone has been able to join and become a member without an access fee.

SOLiD

Invented by Tim Berners Lee (creator of the World Wide Web) and the MIT lab, SOcial LInked Data (SOLiD) is a new framework for the internet that gives users the ability to create granular data sharing agreements. Users can store different types of data in distinct storage spaces: For example, sensitive health or financial information could be saved in the home; whereas, social media data would be in an online cloud. Users can then decide how others access that data, so only authorized organizations, people, or apps can do so.

With SOLiD, every user owns their data, so if an individual becomes dissatisfied with a service, they can just take their data to another site. SOLiD also wants to make data expression standardized, so that diverse data types can be shared by completely different services. By linking user data across different applications, SOLiD aims to achieve a high degree of portability.

As reported by Nesta, SOLiD is young and no major use cases have been developed yet. The team envisions the expansion of the platform being driven in the same way the Apple iStore has grown, by third parties creating their own apps that others will want to use. In the meantime, the SOLiD team has built a series of prototype applications, including a blogging platform, an address book, and a profile editor.

Blockchain/Blockstack

We spent time earlier in the book discussing blockchain, so all we will say here is that in Europe it is called blockstack. It is the same concept of a distributed and public/open digital ledger used to record transactions between two parties efficiently in a verifiable and permanent way that we touched on earlier.

The potential applications for blockchain are seemingly limitless, and the tremendous benefits it could bring cannot be understated. It literally has the potential to become the system of record for all transactions. The strengths of blockchain technology are its security, efficiency, and noncentralized control. In addition to making crypto currencies possible, these strengths could quite easily provide the foundation for a more decentralized internet that puts data ownership back into the hands of users, and where apps run locally rather than from a centralized server.

DECODE

DEcentralized Citizen Owned Data Ecosystem (DECODE) is an experimental project to develop practical alternatives to how we use the internet today by giving people a choice about what happens to their digital identity and who uses their data online for which purposes.

Four European pilots aim to show the wider social value that comes with individuals being given the power to take control of their personal data as well as the means to share their data differently. The pilot projects will include workshops in collaboration with citizens and communities, designing functions that meet specific requirements of the users as well as political and geographical issues related to the host city (Amsterdam and Barcelona).

Make It Easy for Patients to Get Their Own Medical Records

It may be another decade before personal data sovereignty becomes the norm, but in the meantime medical providers should make it easy, fast, and affordable for patients to access and receive copies of their own medical record.

Unfortunately, a recent study published in the *Journal of the American Medical Association* found that patients are often inhibited from accessing their records due to complicated, lengthy, and costly medical records request processes. Despite federal laws that have long promoted patient access to their own medical records, a lack of transparency in the medical records request process as well as a lack of a uniform procedure for requesting medical records make it challenging for many patients to obtain a copy of their medical records from hospitals across the US.

The researchers conducting the study in *JAMA* had difficulty even contacting some hospitals, and for those they did get in touch with, many had no protocol for providing medical records in digital form, despite being required to do so by HIPAA, and when fulfilling hard-copy requests charged patients anywhere from nothing to over $500.

This study makes clear that hospitals have not embraced sharing medical records or creating an easy and convenient way for patients to make the request in the first place. As the authors note, patients want access to their own medical record, and allowing patients to have it results in better patient understanding about their health information, improved care coordination and communication with their physician, and better adherence to treatment. We understand that accessing and printing a medical record can be a challenge, but it isn't that difficult, and it shouldn't cost very much.

Organizations and consumers will both need to come to terms with the new realities of personal data sovereignty. Organizations will need to align with the changing mindsets and desires of consumers when it comes to management of personal data and to evaluate and adapt existing systems to ensure compatibility. They must also be willing to relinquish control of consumer data while they continue to deliver a customer-friendly experience for their users.

On the other hand, consumers will need to be aware of and accept the pros and cons of self-managing their data. Rather than having organizations manage it on their behalf, the burden of managing and allocating access to their own data will be borne by each individual. Further, consumers will have to learn how to view and manage their data as assets they now control.

Fortunately, disruptors are ready to help. Another disruptor highlighted by Nesta, the Tactical Technology Collective (TTC) works in the field of privacy and personal data and combines activism, awareness-raising, and projects that make complex topics more accessible to the general public.

TTC has produced the *Data Detox Kit*, an eight-day guide that helps people work through different aspects of their digital life and to gain more control over it. Its *Trackography* project is an interactive map that shows where one's internet browsing data are moving around the world and which companies have access to it when you access different websites. They've also created *Me and My Shadow*, a website providing resources and how-to guides for navigating today's online, connected world.

The project challenges people to look a little deeper into the settings on their various technologies and to follow simple techniques to protect their privacy.

The aforementioned technologies may pave the road to a future where consumers own their data and where large-scale cyber breaches involving millions of stolen personal identities are a thing of the past. As the GDPR becomes a normal, everyday part of consumers' lives and organizations' practices in Europe, consumers in other parts of the world will demand the same. People will gradually become aware of the need and be increasingly motivated to be protective of their data. Organizations will need to evolve accordingly and bear responsibility for the just use and management of consumer data.

> People will gradually become aware of the need and be **increasingly motivated** to be protective of their data.

The question is how fast can healthcare organizations become compliant with the rules put forth in the EU's General Data Protection Regulation. What can healthcare organizations do to return ownership of consumer data back to consumers? How can healthcare organizations rewrite their privacy policies so they are more easily understood? How can healthcare organizations turn consumer-focused transparency and control into a competitive advantage? They shouldn't wait for the US government to pass a law similar to the GDPR. They shouldn't wait for large employers (many of whom do business in Europe and will themselves be compliant with GDPR) to ask for them to do so. They should just go ahead and do it. Now.

CHAPTER TAKEAWAYS

Earlier chapters addressed what we believe is needed to help healthcare organizations survive. These were near-term tasks necessary to meet the emerging threats to healthcare's current way of business. These were also the steps that will help healthcare leaders get ready for what large employers are already asking for and what increasing numbers of employers and consumers will soon be demanding.

This chapter made suggestions for a few longer-term actions we believe the healthcare industry as a whole should confront. Moving these larger issues—eldercare, the food industry, Big Pharma, and personal data—will require the clout of the entire healthcare industry, but they will go far to improve people's health as well as reduce the cost of care.

5

Doing Major Surgery on Washington: Politicians, **Fix the Mess** You've Created!

THE FREE MARKET IS THE ONLY THING THAT CAN SAVE OUR HEALTHCARE SYSTEM. WE ASK FOR HELP FROM THE GOVERNMENT WITH TREPIDATION.

The US healthcare system desperately needs reform to rein in costs, improve quality, and expand access. This book has focused on what the industry can and should do to transform itself. We've highlighted trailblazers who are driving disruptive innovation, as well as changes driven by employers, savvy medical care providers, and industry leaders who are devising solutions to the problems consumers confront every day in our ailing system.

Our underlying belief is that the healthcare industry must drive the changes needed to repair itself. Furthermore, we're skeptical that needed reforms will come from the government, where politicians, policy experts, and pundits fruitlessly debate how to pay for our ruinously expensive healthcare system rather than finding ways to rein in costs and improve quality. Top-down solutions alone cannot fix such a wasteful and misdirected system; however, several federal policy changes would go a long way to improving healthcare while helping consumers move beyond what the industry itself can do on its own. Debate is ongoing, and there is more nuance to each of them than we capture.

Like anything else, there are good and bad aspects within many of the laws we discuss here. We've taken a higher-level view and presented a streamlined and simplified summary of the existing information. We encourage anyone interested in learning more to pursue some of the in-depth coverage and analysis documented in our Endnotes.

The following topics are addressed in descending order starting with those we believe would have the biggest positive impact on healthcare. These represent a unique and historic opportunity for the US government to save money, save lives, and restore healthcare to something we can be proud of.

CHANGE TAX LAWS RELATED TO EMPLOYER-SPONSORED HEALTH PLANS

The current tax laws regarding employer-sponsored health benefits are an artifact of World War II when the government gave preferential tax treatment to companies that provided health insurance to their employees. At that time this was a way for companies to attract and retain workers in a very tight labor market. It was reasonable and made sense during a world war when wage controls were in place, but the effect of these laws enduring over time has been to prevent people from seeing the direct (and true) costs of healthcare.

The unlimited income exclusion for company-provided health expenses created harmful, counterproductive incentives. It encouraged higher demand for care (regardless of cost) while distorting insurance into covering nearly all services rather than reserving insurance for catastrophic illnesses (like every other form of insurance). Premium subsidies in the Affordable Care Act and the more recent tax credits proposed by the GOP artificially prop up high insurance premiums for bloated coverage that minimizes out-of-pocket payments. This further disconnects people from the actual costs of care, prevents most people from caring about prices, and practically eliminates incentives for the healthcare industry to compete on price.

The tax code can play an important role in realigning consumer incentives to put downward pressure on prices. We believe tax deductions for companies providing health insurance should be eliminated. This will make the tax code less complicated as well as provide the simplest, most efficient pathway to a free market for healthcare. It will also bring health insurance back to the same standard as every other form of insurance (such as homeowners and auto), none of which are paid for by employers or tax deductible.

The tax code can play an important role in realigning consumer incentives to put downward pressure on prices.

If eliminating the tax deduction for companies that provide health insurance to their employees is not politically possible, then individuals who purchase their own health insurance should be given the same preferential tax treatment that companies receive. Furthermore, any tax deductions for money used to purchase health insurance (by companies or individuals) should be capped so they can be used only to purchase catastrophic coverage. This would help reduce counterproductive incentives that ultimately limit consumers' consideration of the value of medical care.

Increased competition from consumers' comparison shopping in the individual market would drive down premiums. Workers would have many more insurance policy options, and employers would be freed from the ever-growing cost and frustration of administering health benefits.

EXPAND HEALTH SAVINGS ACCOUNTS

Health savings accounts (known as HSAs) are tax-advantaged savings vehicles that allow consumers to set aside money to pay for health-related expenses. Pretax money is contributed to an HSA, thereby reducing overall taxable income for federal and state taxation. HSA funds can be used to pay for qualified medical expenses at any time without federal tax liability or penalty.

HSAs are currently available only to US consumers who are enrolled in high-deductible health plans. In 2019 the amount a person can contribute to an HSA is $3,500 for an individual and $7,000 for a family, and this is adjusted upward annually to account for inflation. Anyone over fifty-five can contribute an additional $1,000 annually.

Once you're over age sixty-five and enrolled in Medicare, you can no longer contribute to an HSA, but you can still use the money in an HSA for out-of-pocket medical expenses. If the money is used on noneligible expenses, you will have to pay income tax on that amount (plus a penalty if you're under sixty-five).

Unlike a flexible spending account (FSA), HSA funds roll over and accumulate year to year if they are not spent, so people do not have to worry about losing any savings. HSAs are an important tool that can help reduce the growth of healthcare costs and increase the efficiency of the healthcare system. HSAs encourage saving for future healthcare expenses, allow consumers to receive the care they want and are willing to pay for, and push consumers to be more responsible for their own healthcare choices.

To move toward the ideal future of consumer-centric healthcare, Congress should pass legislation making HSAs universally available to all Americans (including seniors on Medicare) so long as they have some form of health insurance (not necessarily a high-deductible health plan). Higher contribution limits should also be set in recognition of the increasing costs of medical care as people age. In addition, restrictions on the use of HSA funds should be reduced to allow payment for care of elderly parents as well as for one's own long-term care.

RATIONALIZE HEALTHCARE SUBSIDIES

Those of us who have worked in healthcare have often thought the whole payment system to be an absolute mess. One CEO was heard saying to some administrators and physicians he had invited to a poker game, "Be sure and bring real money, not those crazy healthcare dollars."

The modern healthcare system is built on cross-subsidy. Generally speaking, commercial health insurers such as Blue Cross Blue Shield, Aetna, and Humana pay the highest level of reimbursement to hospitals and medical providers. Medicare pays less than these commercial insurers, while Medicaid reimburses at even lower levels. Hence, commercial payers are charged more to make up for the fact that Medicare and Medicaid pay less than what hospitals charge for their services (remember that most healthcare providers do not know their actual costs). Irrational as it seems, this has been going on for a long time.

Hospital administrators were always looking at their payer mix. Hospitals that make the most money and have the best margins are often the ones that have more commercial payers (such as Blue Cross or Cigna). They are the fortunate ones. As mentioned earlier in this book, however, even these lucky hospitals are beginning to feel the pinch as 10,000 baby boomers a day move from being covered by private insurance to being covered under Medicare. That's 3.65 million a year—a number that is projected to continue until 2030.

The cost of healthcare is difficult to fix because of these types of arrangements, known as cross-subsidies. In a *Wall Street Journal* article written on July 29, 2018, John Cochrane called them the "original sin." He said, "The government wants to subsidize healthcare for poor people, chronically sick people and even people who have money but chose to spend less of it on healthcare than officials find sufficient. These are worthy goals, easily achieved in a completely free-market system by raising taxes and then subsidizing healthcare or insurance, at market prices, for the people the government wishes to help."

Cochrane continued, "But lawmakers don't want to be seen as taxing and spending, so they hide these transfers in cross-subsidies. They require emergency rooms (very expensive) to treat everyone who comes along, and then hospitals must overcharge everyone else."

Add to this the fact that many people who end up in the emergency room might not have gone there in the first place if they had received appropriate primary care. And, as already stated, hospitals overcharge commercial payers and the few patients who pay cash to subsidize Medicare and Medicaid patients.

Cochrane suggests this is done because it doesn't show up on the federal budget but meets the goals of subsidizing healthcare for the poor and chronically sick. He further stated, "Over the long term, cross-subsidies are far more inefficient than forthright taxing and spending. If the hospital is going to overcharge private insurance and paying customers to cross-subsidize the poor, uninsured, Medicare and Medicaid, then the hospital must be protected from the competition. If competitors can come in and offer services to the paying customers, the scheme unravels."

Cochrane compares the current situation in healthcare to telephone and airline service prior to deregulation in the late 1970s. Back then the government forced the phone company (there was only one phone company at the time) to subsidize landlines with overpriced long-distance service, but allowed it to have a monopoly to prevent competition and keep new entrants out of the market.

Similarly, the government forced the airlines to subsidize flights to/from small towns with overpriced flights to/from bigger cities while enforcing an oligopoly to keep new airlines from undercutting the profitable segments. Cochrane notes that "after deregulation, everyone's phone bills and airfares were lower and service was better and more innovative."

We agree with Cochrane and think this kind of deregulation will have the same useful effects on healthcare, and we want competition. Without it there is no pressure to innovate for better service and lower cost. Without competition, everyone pays more than they would in a competitive free market, which is where the US healthcare system has been for some time.

> **"Lack of competition,** especially from new entrants, is the screaming problem in health-care delivery today..."

As Cochrane pointed out, "Lack of competition, especially from new entrants, is the screaming problem in health-care delivery today. In no competitive business will they not tell you the cost before providing service. In a competitive business you are bombarded with ads from new companies offering a better deal." We agree this is exactly what healthcare desperately needs.

ELIMINATE CERTIFICATE OF NEED LAWS

Certificate of need (CON) laws drive up healthcare costs by restricting construction of new medical facilities. According to Dr. Hal Scherz, an Atlanta urologist, "Certificate of need laws are a remnant of a failed theory of government healthcare planning." He further stated, "Their only purpose today is to restrict competition and protect the big hospitals' local monopolies. The federal government, which played a central role in creating this problem, could help solve it by making Medicaid block grants contingent on repeal of certificate of need laws."

Big hospital associations in certificate of need states claim that limiting competition improves access to care. But according to the Mercatus Center at George Mason University, the quality of care in these states is worse. In particular, deaths from treatable complications following surgery and mortality from heart failure, pneumonia, and heart attacks are higher in the states with such laws on the books.

We have stated that to reduce cost and improve quality, care has to be moved to the most appropriate site. These laws prevent that from happening and need to be repealed or healthcare costs will continue to rise.

According to a Mercatus Center working paper, certificate of need laws for MRI, CT, and PET scans exist in twenty-one states. These laws, similar to CON laws for other services, mandate approval processes for scanning technology. One argument for CON laws is that they benefit the patient by keeping healthcare costs low, which they are supposed to do by preventing overinvestment in technology and capital. But according to Mercatus, common-sense economics suggests CON laws restrict competition and set up barriers to entry into healthcare.

The current state-based iteration of CON laws requires hospitals and other facilities to pay an application cost, which averages $32,000 per application (to obtain a CON) but can go up to as high as $5 million in some cases. The fees alone are often enough to prevent all but the large, established players from even trying to open a new facility.

Using data from the American Health Planning Association and the Centers for Medicare and Medicaid Services, Thomas Stratmann and Mathew Baker performed a study about the true effects of CON laws that regulate MRI, CT, and PET scanners. They concluded the following:

> » These laws have a substantial effect on new hospitals and nonhospital providers, but close to no effect on incumbent hospitals.

» Fewer scans of all types are provided in states with CON laws, and the effect is distributed unevenly across provider types.

» There are winners (incumbent hospitals) and losers (potential new entrants) in terms of market share.

» Patients travel farther from their county of residence to obtain care in CON states than in non-CON states.

» CON laws can be barriers in the healthcare industry and they do not benefit patients, as is commonly argued.

Interestingly, one of the reasons incumbent hospitals want CON laws is that they can charge more for services they provide if they can keep competitors out. Researchers found that rates were 15.3 percent higher, on average, in areas with one hospital, compared with those serviced by four or more. In markets with two hospitals, prices were 6.4 percent higher. Where there were three hospitals competing, the prices were only 4.8 percent higher.

Researchers at the Mercatus Center at George Mason University have studied the negative consequences of CON laws. One analysis by Christopher Koopman and Thomas Stratmann found that CON laws in Virginia "could mean approximately 10,800 fewer hospital beds, 41 fewer hospitals offering MRI services, and 58 fewer hospitals offering CT scans." The authors conclude, "this means less competition and fewer choices, without increased access to care for the poor."

USE EVIDENCE-BASED GUIDELINES TO REDUCE THE COMPLIANCE BURDEN

In 2000, Dr. Oliver Schein (an ophthalmologist from Johns Hopkins) and colleagues published a study in the *New England Journal of Medicine* that sought to determine whether routine preoperative medical testing performed in patients scheduled to undergo cataract surgery helped reduce the incidence of intraoperative and postoperative medical complications. Their conclusion was that such routine medical testing before cataract surgery does not measurably increase the safety of the surgery.

Flash forward to a 2017 article in which Dr. Peter Pronovost (a practicing anesthesiologist, critical-care physician, and professor at Johns Hopkins) reported that cataract patients continue to receive testing as part of a preoperative medical exam despite strong evidence that neither the testing nor exam reduce surgical risk.

Pronovost made it clear that requiring the preoperative exam makes sense for the vast majority of surgical procedures since patients may have a host of complicating factors (including multiple conditions, allergies, and complex medication regimens) that could impact their surgery. In those cases, preoperative exams help the surgical team identify and mitigate risks for potential surgical complications.

However, those risks rarely exist in cataract surgery. Pronovost estimated that the cost of these mandatory yet unhelpful exams was roughly half a billion dollars annually (just for cataract patients). He also pointed out that among Medicare patients, no procedure is performed more than cataract surgery, which is projected to grow to 3.3 million surgeries a year by 2020.

Preoperative exams continue to be required by the federal government and accrediting organizations before every cataract operation as well as for many other low-risk elective procedures. Pronovost acknowledged the important role regulations play in ensuring safety for patients and medical staff, but suggested that reducing or eliminating many healthcare regulations, if looked at more closely, could help reduce costs while preserving or even improving safety. For example, Pronovost pointed out that it is more convenient and less expensive for otherwise healthy patients to get long-term intravenous antibiotics at home rather than extend their hospital stay. But Medicare won't cover it.

Pronovost sees encouraging signs that regulators are paying attention. He stated that the Centers for Medicare & Medicaid Services (CMS) "recently removed a regulation that prevented nutritionists from writing diet orders rather than requiring a physician. The decision is expected to save hundreds of millions of dollars and physician time. Yet there are many issues like this that need to be remedied, representing billions of dollars in potential savings."

We agree with Pronovost, who recommended that "CMS should establish a process to identify, evaluate and revise or remove regulations that corset clinicians, increase costs and place burdens on patients without clear benefits to safety or quality."

SIMPLIFY CREDENTIALING AND REMOVE OUTMODED SCOPE-OF-PRACTICE LIMITS

Earlier in our book we alluded to a projected shortage of physicians in this country, which ranged from 40,000 to over 120,000 physicians. We also stated our belief that the physician shortage could be mitigated by moving work to the most appropriate skill set and the most appropriate care setting.

Physicians readily admit they are often working at the lower end of their skill set by performing tasks that others with less training could do just as well. Our book is all about introducing free-market forces into the healthcare arena. When this happens, there will be added pressure to redesign the system to provide more care at less cost, and physicians will, by necessity, be repurposed to handle the more complicated patients while midlevel and other highly skilled but less expensive healthcare resources take care of people in need of less complicated care.

...the government should eliminate archaic obstacles to competition among medical providers...

To facilitate this, the government should eliminate archaic obstacles to competition among medical providers so patients have options to seek the best value for their money. That means simplifying the credentialing requirements and removing out-moded scope-of-practice limits on qualified nurse practitioners and physician assistants. Private clinics staffed by these professionals can provide less expensive primary care.

In a 2011 review, 88 percent of visits to retail clinics involved simple care, which is 30 to 40 percent less expensive than care provided at physicians' offices and about 80 percent less expensive than emergency departments. Interestingly, it comes with high levels of patient satisfaction.

REDUCE RESTRICTIONS ON PHYSICIAN TRAINING

The Social Security Act of 1965 mandated that a portion of Medicare would cover residency costs of physician training. However, the Balanced Budget Act of 1997 capped the number of most physician residencies to the unweighted number of residencies on a teaching hospital's most recent report. At the time, Congress said it would revisit the residency cap, but it never has, so the cap remains and has stymied needed increases in residency training and created a bottleneck for both primary care and specialist physicians.

As another way to help mitigate the potential physician shortage, the US Congress should lift the cap on federally funded residency training positions. Congress should also consider expanding other programs such as the Conrad 30 Waiver Program for immigrant doctors, the National Health Service Corps and Public Service Loan Forgiveness, and Title VII/VIII to recruit a diverse workforce and encourage physicians to practice in shortage specialties and underserved communities.

The bottom line is that residency limits reduce the supply of physicians, artificially restrict competition, and should be publicly scrutinized. Finally, national physician licensing should replace nonreciprocal state licensing. This will go far in preventing unsafe physicians from moving from one state to another to keep practicing and will facilitate the spread of high-quality interstate telemedicine.

ADOPT THE EU'S GENERAL DATA PROTECTION REGULATION

We mentioned that the European Union has gotten in front of the data sovereignty megatrend with the implementation of the General Data Protection Regulation (GDPR), which took effect on May 25, 2018. Designed to modernize laws that protect the personal information of individuals, these regulations give European citizens easier access to the data companies hold about them, more control over what data organizations can collect about them, how they collect it, and what it is used for. Citizens can also demand to see what data are held on them and request that their personal data be deleted.

The GDPR also places obligations on organizations that handle data relating to EU citizens, even if they are based outside the EU. These obligations include protecting this information and being transparent about how it is going to be used. Any organization wanting to do business in the EU will have to comply with the GDPR or face significant fines.

We believe there is absolutely no reason for any organization anywhere in the free world to wait any longer and that they should simply adopt the GDPR and make it their default standard for customer data and privacy. The healthcare industry should advocate for and take the lead in giving consumers complete control over their digital lives, at least as it pertains to their health and health records.

With respect to medical records, they should belong to patients—not to providers, hospitals, or insurers—and they should go with patients wherever they are. We're also realists and believe most US companies will wait for the government to pass similar legislation. So in the best interests of its citizens, the federal government should adopt the EU's General Data Protection Regulation.

CHAPTER TAKEAWAYS

Our underlying belief is that the healthcare industry must drive the changes needed to repair itself. Furthermore, we believe reforms made by the government will not be enough to save healthcare. While politicians, policy experts, and pundits fruitlessly debate how to pay for our ruinously expensive healthcare system, they have consistently failed to rein in costs and improve quality. In fact, it is sometimes easy to throw up our hands and agree with Will Rogers who once said, "Be thankful you're not getting all of the government you're paying for."

Having said that, we described several federal policy changes in this chapter we believe would go a long way toward improving healthcare while helping consumers beyond what the industry itself can do on its own.

6

A Discharge Summary and Glimpse into the **Future of Healthcare**

THE FUTURE BELONGS TO THOSE
WHO WILL SEIZE THEIR DREAM,
WITH COURAGE AND LOVE IN
THEIR HEARTS FOR THOSE THEY
ARE CALLED TO SERVE.

We opened this book with a request that you imagine, with us, the ideal healthcare system of the future. It would look like this:

» Imagine a different mindset for health and healthcare in the United States.

» Imagine that health and well-being are lifelong pursuits for individuals.

» Imagine a true healthcare system that delivers solutions to improve health—not just treat/manage disease.

» Imagine a healthcare system that addresses patients' physical, social, and emotional circumstances as well as basic resource needs (such as food and shelter) as a routine part of care.

» Imagine that evidence-based information about which diagnostics and therapies work best and how much they cost are readily available to individuals and caregivers whenever it is needed.

» Imagine that this evidence-based information includes both traditional and alternative methods.

» Imagine a healthcare system that does not center on doctors, hospitals, and drug/device manufacturers. Instead, it centers on consumers and their families who are fully capable of making decisions about their health needs because they are provided with the necessary tools, information, and opportunity.

When it comes to disruption, healthcare is a paradox in several ways. First, it is both fast and slow. While breakthroughs in life-altering medical treatments seem to come forth at a torrid pace, innovations in the way healthcare is actually delivered happen glacially.

Second, healthcare delivery is split in half with regard to effectiveness. In responding to acute diseases and emergencies, healthcare shows brilliant results. But it simultaneously lags behind in keeping people healthy and when dealing with chronic degenerative conditions such as heart disease, diabetes, and obesity.

Third, consumer surveys have shown that two in three people remain dissatisfied with healthcare costs and access to insurance, while three in four are satisfied with its quality of care. But no one is happy with the industry's dismal record of "doing no harm."

Although disruption by its very nature isn't linear—and that's especially true in healthcare, where disruptions have come sporadically—overall the pace of change is accelerating. And in an industry this big, this important, and this expansive, disruption will continue unabated.

The established healthcare business model is justifiably under assault, and our intent was to help healthcare leaders reframe it by painting a picture of truly consumer/patient–centric healthcare. In the preceding chapters we outlined the risks healthcare leaders face and described specific things they can do in the short and long term to disrupt the industry before someone else (like Amazon, Walmart, or Boeing) does.

We hope you picked up on a few core changes in how healthcare will be viewed and delivered. We are in a transition from a mindset of sickness to a proclivity toward wellness. We are moving from an environment where consumers are frequently kept in the dark to a mindset where consumers should be enlightened. In addition, we are shifting the focus from treatment to prevention, from a reactive to a more proactive model, and from episodic care to a more holistic approach where the health of people will be a key indicator of success for the industry.

Several key themes are emerging from everything that is happening. These trends underscore the need for disruptive innovation in healthcare and should guide your efforts moving forward.

KEY THEME #1:
CONSUMER CENTRIC

Consumers are fed up with the current healthcare system and disappointed with many aspects of it. Even simple tasks such as updating a prescription or requesting a routine appointment have become overly complicated, time-consuming, and inconvenient.

Unlike in every other industry, consumers and patients do not come first in healthcare. In fact, the interests of hospitals, insurers, doctors, drug manufacturers, and other industry players nearly always supersede those of consumers and patients.

In addition, consumers and patients are becoming increasingly responsible for paying the costs of their own care and are beginning to shop around (at least with the slowly increasing number of free-market providers who are willing to post their prices).

At the same time, consumers have become accustomed to doing an increasing array of activities easily and instantly through various technologies (such as staying current with news, communicating with each other, shopping, banking, and paying bills). Today's technology-based conveniences are quickly being taken for granted by many, and consumers increasingly expect fast, sophisticated services and products that cater to their needs.

A number of disruptive innovators see the growing discontent among consumers and employers regarding healthcare. Fueled by their own direct experience with healthcare's shortcomings, they are actively questioning the industry's existing paradigms and attempting to fundamentally change the system, so it is much more consumer centric. Their efforts will enable consumers to easily access the information necessary to make informed choices about health and medical care.

Consumer decisions will be based on meaningful comparative data, not on a physician's or hospital's general reputation, the experiences of friends, or where a physician has admitting privileges. Consumers will know exactly what each physician and hospital charges for standard procedures and what their bill will be when they make a choice. Consumers will also know the quality scores and safety outcomes for each physician and hospital.

With this information, consumers will be empowered, able, and financially incented to seek out the most cost-effective care with the best outcomes without worrying about whether a provider is in or out of network. They will choose the most affordable care with the best outcomes. Like every other industry, medical providers will truly compete for consumers' business.

KEY THEME #2:
EMPLOYER DRIVEN

Incumbent companies in various industries are beginning to disrupt healthcare by taking interesting and creative approaches to the way they provide health coverage for their employees. Although Amazon, Apple, and Google are receiving the most attention, many other employers are aggressively trying to rein in their health costs. Every company is doing something to control their healthcare costs, but a growing number and variety of organizations are beginning to fundamentally change how they view the health of their workforce as well as the provision of healthcare to them.

Largely due to frustration with incessantly rising costs, some large companies are discarding long-held practices and adopting a do-it-yourself approach. These innovative companies are moving toward empowering staff by providing support and assistance to help them make better decisions for themselves and their families regarding health and healthcare. These organizations have turned to independent services to help employees navigate the fragmented and confusing healthcare marketplace.

The underlying precept for these organizations is that the focus should be on employee health and wellness. They also believe employees should not feel alone, confused, or overwhelmed when it comes to understanding and choosing healthcare. In addition, a few companies have partnered directly with health vendors to provide services to their staff and their family members, bypassing traditional health insurance plans altogether.

Disruption in healthcare will be driven by innovative organizations like Walmart, Boeing, Comcast, and others. These and other employers will do more to stimulate competition among healthcare providers and increase the supply of medical care to the people of the United States than the government could ever imagine.

KEY THEME #3:
FREE MARKET AND COMPETITION

Our current healthcare system does not operate like anything resembling a free market, where consumers are in control and can easily shop around for the medical providers who deliver the best service and outcomes at the most reasonable prices. Medical providers have a perplexing array of prices for any given service/procedure, which are seemingly not tethered to any form of reality. Prices seem arbitrary, and sometimes predatory, with little oversight and no market incentive to reduce them.

Besides gambling, healthcare is the only industry where consumers are forced to make major decisions in ignorance of, and often against, their own economic interests. Many consumers don't realize a procedure can cost two to three times more at different hospitals, are unaware of how much is really being spent, and have little incentive to know the underlying costs.

Consumers attempting to price compare will find it extremely difficult and time-consuming to get any healthcare provider to commit to a firm price. And those who do take advantage of price comparisons available through various websites will find the preposterously expansive price ranges surrealistic.

Innovative organizations like Walmart, Boeing, Comcast, and others are forcing medical providers to assume much, if not all, of the risk for the health of their employee populations. They are demanding price guarantees and are willing to fly employees across the country to undergo procedures in centers of excellence where the care is better and the prices are up to 50 percent less. They view this as an important way to reduce healthcare costs. These employers are also taking steps to empower and incent their employees to seek value. Collectively, they are creating the conditions in which a more market-oriented healthcare system will emerge.

KEY THEME #4:
HEALTH AND WELLNESS INSTEAD
OF JUST SICK CARE

Unhealthy behaviors such as poor eating habits, lack of exercise, and smoking cost this country an estimated $1.5 billion each year in the treatment of preventable conditions such as heart disease, cancer, lung diseases, and diabetes. But as our healthcare system gains proficiency in treating chronic diseases, Americans struggle to modify behaviors that contribute to these diseases in the first place. Despite the plethora of evidence buttressing the importance of prevention as a way to save lives and money, the majority of our healthcare spending is directed toward treating (often preventable) illnesses.

The high-tech disruptors who are often in the news (Amazon, Apple, and Google) and other innovative employers are focusing on reducing healthcare costs by helping their own employees with better prevention and wellness. They are primarily thinking about employee health and join the 80 percent of employers who offer preventive and wellness services to their staff.

They also recognize the role wellness can play in keeping their workforce healthy, engaged, and productive. The better employee wellness programs also include elements to account for and connect other factors that impact people's wellness, happiness, and life. In addition to physical wellness, these other components include financial, emotional, and social wellness.

Employers and consumers increasingly recognize that to optimize a person's physical well-being, it is necessary to understand how the different components of wellness influence one another, and to address all of them. The healthcare system of the future will deliver solutions to improve health—not just treat/manage disease. It will also address patients' physical, social, and emotional circumstances as well as basic resource needs (such as food and shelter) as a routine part of care. Because people will become more responsible for their own medical costs, health and well-being will become lifelong pursuits for more and more people.

KEY THEME #5:
IDEAS ENHANCED BY TECHNOLOGY

Cutting-edge technologies have played a prominent role in the disruption of other industries. Think of Amazon, PayPal, Netflix, Uber, Airbnb, Facebook, and many others. Undoubtedly, new technologies will play a prominent role in the forthcoming disruption in healthcare. These will come in the form of better and more targeted drugs, 3-D printed organs, smart/integrated electronic medical records, the use of virtual reality to help patients heal as well as help them pass the time while recovering, and many others. But purely technological disruptions represent just a fraction of the changes that will occur in healthcare.

In many other areas (such as telemedicine, home care, artificial intelligence augmentation for healthcare providers), new technologies will play an enabling role rather than a driving role. These technologies will augment providers, help move care closer to those who need it, and reduce the cost of care. Augmentation technologies will improve testing and diagnostic capabilities and will shift work to the appropriate level (in other words, enabling primary care physicians, nurses, and even self-care practitioners with some level of training to do work once performed by specialists).

Many disruptors have seemingly found a better way to do something through technology. But a closer look shows that it wasn't the technology that elevated them into prominence, but a different mindset.

Disruption will occur and cause a painful struggle for hospitals, medical providers, and the broader healthcare industry. The intensity of the pain will depend on whether the healthcare delivery system disrupts itself or if others disrupt it.

John Dewey said, "Every great advance in science has issued from a new audacity of imagination." Therefore, the trials that lie ahead will be difficult, but are not insurmountable. Leaders in other industries, especially those who have already experienced disruption, will have little sympathy as they rightly believe healthcare should have done this a long time ago—and saved them billions of dollars in healthcare costs.

LOOKING AHEAD

In spite of the struggles that lie ahead for the healthcare delivery system, we think it is a great and very exciting time to be alive. Creating the ideal future state for healthcare will require imagination and insight as well as an obsessive focus on consumers. In the end the wellness and healthcare system will be transformed to be accessible to more people at higher quality and at much less cost. New and exciting experiments, ideas, concepts, and products seem to be popping up everywhere.

For example, in just a recent two-week period, we have heard or read the following:

» That the USDA food pyramid we have all been taught since childhood is excellent for fattening cattle. This is not new to many of us, but we had never heard it put that way.

» That healthy fat is much better as fuel for the body and brain than sugar and refined carbohydrates. Talk about a paradigm shift. This is explained clearly in the book *The Ketogenic Reset Diet* by Mark Sisson. It is sweeping the nation and may be just a fad, but makes a lot of sense when you read Sisson's book.

» That people who exercise may be exercising way too much since recovery time is the most important part of your exercise program. This is new, at least to most of us, but the evidence is mounting in support of this thinking.

» That virtual reality is being used to treat smokers, alcoholics, and crack addicts; in teaching medical students; and in making life better for the elderly in retirement homes. It is also a lot of fun. If you haven't tried it, you should.

» That psychedelic drugs in micro doses, combined with therapy, are being successfully used by major universities to treat PTSD, depression, and addiction to cigarettes, and a variety of other conditions.

» That taking prebiotics is better than just taking probiotics because there are healthy and unhealthy microbes in the body. When fed prebiotics, the healthy microbes grow, and the unhealthy ones diminish.

» That much of what we have been told by the healthcare community over the years is wrong. See *Lies My Doctor Told Me: Medical Myths That Can Harm Your Health* by Dr. Ken D. Berry.

» That going barefoot outside in the grass and getting fifteen to twenty minutes of sunshine a day is great for your mitochondria, which are essential to your health.

» That we are mostly just energy with hardly any matter at all. In fact, if all of the actual matter of all the humans on the earth were combined, it would be the size of a sugar cube. And we have barely scratched the surface of the possibilities understanding this will bring to the wellness and healthcare community. (We know this sounds strange, so we recommend you read the rather amazing book, *Reality Unveiled* by Ziad Masri.)

And so forth…all in just two weeks of health news! It is all a bit overwhelming, but also extremely exciting.

The next section is called "For Further Information." In the first part entitled "Disruptive Organizations within Healthcare," we have outlined many of the amazing forces, products, services, and businesses that are currently disrupting healthcare. Be sure to have your disruptive innovation teams review this information as they start disrupting your organization and designing new forms of care. We think you will find it very helpful.

A second part, "Disruptive Organizations Outside of Healthcare," is equally interesting and potentially useful for your design teams. As the title implies, we have outlined disruptive activity found in the nonhealthcare space but that might stimulate new thinking as well.

As we look to the future, we see exciting, maybe even unimaginable possibilities because innovative people are never satisfied with the status quo. They constantly ask, "What if?" and "Why not?" They challenge conventional wisdom and disrupt things to make them better.

We believe the most important step that should be taken to reshape the healthcare delivery system is to make it more—not less—human. It is easy to get enraptured with new technologies, methods, relationships, and communities. But the guiding lights for all of this should be less need for care, improved care and caring when needed, reduced cost, reduced risks, more access, and greater ease of use by the customer.

No one can really predict the future of medicine, but if we can hold to these guidelines and constantly and respectfully listen to our customers, there is hope we will not go too far astray.

Another point to emphasize is that sustaining innovation alone, while necessary, is insufficient. Healthcare leaders can easily make the mistake of focusing only on the new and exciting technologies, products, and methodologies. But customers will still be demanding more access and less expensive care.

So healthcare leaders shouldn't fail to disrupt their organizations to meet this demand, perhaps along the lines of what Iora Health and others have done, or they may not have an organization that can enjoy all of the new technologies.

Finally, just a brief scanning of this chapter should give any sentient being the impression that things are changing and changing rapidly. Innovation seems to be moving at breakneck speed, taking your breath away. Ignore at your own peril. We have made suggestions regarding how to change organizational culture to engage more minds, think more creatively, experiment constantly, and learn ever more rapidly.

We do not suggest that the healthcare industry panic. We think there is still time, but the clock is ticking and everyone in healthcare should start this exciting journey sooner rather than later. There is much to do. We hope this book will help you move forward.

FOR FURTHER INFORMATION

DISRUPTIVE ORGANIZATIONS WITHIN HEALTHCARE

The newest generation of healthcare disruptors are pursuing wildly different goals in unique ways but have several goals in common—to empower people, increase engagement, enhance satisfaction, produce better health outcomes, and lower healthcare costs. Most of the disruptors use technology as a foundational element of their products or services to empower and serve customers, but some function as diagnostic or informational tools while others provide physical products or services.

Here we highlight particularly innovative disruptors within the healthcare space, organized by the type of service they provide.

Healthcare Delivery

» Centene – A multi-line managed care enterprise that serves as a major intermediary for both government-sponsored and privately insured healthcare programs. Centene also contracts with other healthcare and commercial organizations to provide specialty services, including behavioral healthcare services, case management software, in-home health services, life and health management, vision, pharmacy benefits management, and telehealth services. Centene accomplishes their goal of transforming the community, one person at a time, by helping people adopt healthy lifestyles to enhance wellness, minimize sickness, and reduce the need for expensive acute care services.

» Narayana Health – Offers globally benchmarked, quality-driven, and affordable healthcare. Implementation of the latest technologies, such as using tablets in the ICU instead of patient charts, simulation technology to help train critical-care nurses, and telemedicine for those in remote parts of India, has helped to deliver a far higher quality of healthcare that's helping to keep patients safer and create better recovery outcomes. This system includes a cardiac care hospital, a cancer care hospital (the largest in India), a women's and children's hospital, along with nephrology, orthopedic, and research and training centers. With twenty-six hospitals in sixteen cities built over a fifteen-year period, their vision is to further develop 30,000 beds in the next seven years in newly built hospitals across India and the Cayman Islands.

TeleMedicine–Virtual Care

» Aiva Health – A voice-powered care assistant that uses smart speakers like Amazon Alexa and Google Home to connect patients and seniors with their care providers. Both Amazon and Google have invested in Aiva.

» Akira – A mobile app that lets customers connect instantly with a team of doctors and nurse practitioners. Users can text or video chat as much as they like.

» American Well – An online and mobile telehealth company that connects patients instantly with doctors over secure video. The company also provides immediate urgent care web visits for patients in forty-six states.

» Doctor on Demand – A web service that provides a fast and easy way to get care from physicians. The online visit allows patients to connect within minutes through a live video visit with a board-certified primary care physician from nearly any mobile device, while at home, in the workplace, or while traveling.

» HealthTap – A mobile app that lets customers connect immediately or by appointment to over 107,000 doctors via videoconference, text chats, or phone call 24/7 for free. An AI-powered "physician" routes/triages customers to the right level of care at the right time based on the patient's symptoms.

» Grand Rounds – A company that connects patients with local and remote specialty care via phone, web, mobile application, and text chat. Grand Rounds offers two major services: office visits and expert opinions. The first service identifies the top local experts for both surgical and nonsurgical specialties based on quantitative analysis, while the second connects consumers' local physicians with remote specialists for a collaborative team approach to tough cases.

Promoting Evidence-Based Medicine

» Cochrane Collaboration – an international independent and not-for-profit organization dedicated to making up-to-date, accurate information about the effects of healthcare readily available worldwide. It produces and disseminates systematic reviews of healthcare interventions and promotes the search for evidence in the form of clinical trials and other studies of interventions.

» Consumers United for Evidence-based Healthcare (CUE) – a national coalition of health and consumer advocacy organizations committed to empowering consumers to make the best use of evidence-based healthcare.

» RightCare Alliance – a grassroots coalition of healthcare professionals, patients, and community groups that seeks to counter the trend of increasing medical costs that don't add value to patients by helping them avoid treatments that research has shown are ineffective or even dangerous.

Medical Treatments

» Levita Magnetics – A company that has developed a new system that uses magnets in a novel way—to retract and maneuver organs—with a goal of making it possible for surgeons to perform single port surgery for common abdominal procedures such as gall bladder removals and appendectomies. Levita Magnetics intends to be a catalyst in the continued evolution of less invasive surgery.

» Mdacne – A mobile app with the goal of making dermatology more accessible, convenient, and affordable. Consumers take a selfie in a well-lit room using the Mdacne app. In a matter of seconds, the app's advanced computer vision technology analyzes the consumer's skin and provides a full analysis of their skin condition, free of charge. The company will then send a fully customized acne treatment kit with products formulated to treat the consumer's unique skin condition.

» Not Impossible Labs – An incubator and content studio dedicated to changing the world through technology and story. Not Impossible Labs has engineered, programmed, hacked, and crowd-solved issues of inability and inaccessibility and provided low-cost solutions for the most vulnerable on our planet. Current projects include creating a nonpharmaceutical therapy to improve motor systems disrupted by Parkinson's, using mobile technology to create a network to reduce hunger among those struggling with food insecurity, a wearable allowing young children losing their hearing or vision to better traverse the world around them.

» Range of Motion Project (ROMP) – A nonprofit, for-impact healthcare organization dedicated to providing prosthetic and orthotic care to those without access to these services. ROMP refurbishes donated components, purchases new components, and even invents components to get patients what they need.

Pharmacy Services

» PillPack – A full-service, online pharmacy that delivers a better, simpler experience for people who manage multiple medications through convenient packaging and personalized service. Each month, customers receive a personalized roll of presorted medications, along with a convenient dispenser and any other medications that cannot be placed into packets, like liquids and inhalers. Each shipment includes a medication label that has a picture of each pill and notes on how it should be taken. PillPack manages each customer's medications, coordinates refills and renewals, and makes sure each shipment is sent on time, every time. PillPack also enables real-time notifications and an online dashboard so customers can control their shipments, refills, and copays. Note: Amazon purchased PillPack in June 2018 for nearly $1 billion.

» CareZone Pharmacy – An online pharmacy that delivers medications to the consumer's home, free of charge. Customers receive convenient presorted pill packets organized by dosage, date, and time. Simply tear open a pack for exact medications needed. The mobile app also enables users to manage their medications and refills.

Medical Testing–Diagnostics

» AliveCor Kardia Mobile – A secure mobile app that lets consumers receive a medical-grade EKG in thirty seconds, enabling users to know anytime, anywhere if their heart rhythm is normal or if atrial fibrillation is detected. Results are delivered to users' smartphones.

» GlowDX – Uses DNA-computing technology to create a fast, easy-to-use, and inexpensive diagnostic tool for dengue fever and other tropical diseases in the developing world. GlowDX is currently developing a point-of-care platform to bring a fully integrated sample preparation and molecular diagnostic system to those who need it most for launch in 2021.

» Dreem – A sleep monitoring headband that discreetly records and analyzes brain activity, movement, heart rate, and respiration. The system synchronizes with the customer's brain activity in real time and uses sound via bone conduction technology to improve one's sleep quality.

Personal Behavior Modification

» NextHealth Technologies – A technology platform that enables health insurers to sift through client data to identify patients with the greatest opportunity for change. The company uses analytics to determine the best manner to reach those people—a phone call, mailer, text message, email, or combination—with important information, advice, reminders. NextHealth then analyzes millions of claims to determine if its communication altered patient behavior. If not, it tries another strategy. Over time, NextHealth learns individuals' preferences, just as Google does.

» Optimity – A mobile app with gamified wellness solutions that uses a data-driven approach to prevent employees from becoming sick. The technology enables a strategic approach to preventive wellness through holistic content, micro-habits or small daily actions woven into people's existing routines, and social support from friends and colleagues.

» Omada – A digital behavior change program that can help people lose weight, reduce their risk for chronic disease, and feel better. The program uses behavior science to guide participants through an inspiring and interactive journey that integrates seamlessly into everyday life. The intent is to help people change their habits, improve their health, and reduce their risk of chronic disease.

» Upright Go – A digital behavior change program for better posture and improved well-being. Upright Go is a biofeedback trainer that uses a small wearable device that alerts people to improve their posture simply by vibrating every time they slouch.

» Propeller Health – A digital platform for management of chronic conditions such as asthma and COPD. Through sensors, mobile apps, and services, Propeller helps reduce the cost of care while delivering better quality of life for individuals with chronic respiratory disease.

Personal Health Enhancement

» Headspace – A company that provides guided meditation online, accessible to its registered users through the company's website and mobile app with the goal of mindfulness. Headspace has been used in a number of clinical trials investigating the effects of mindfulness training. One such trial found a significant increase in well-being, reductions in anxiety and depressive symptoms, significant reductions in diastolic blood pressures, significant increases in perceived job control, as well as a significant reduction in sleeping problems. It also helps in significantly reducing stress in the mind and the body.

» Virta – An empirically based, ketogenic diet program with a smartphone app for daily monitoring by physicians and dietary coaches, video-based learning, shared community, and a track record of getting 80 percent of their type 2 diabetic patients completely off meds.

Genetic Testing

» 23andMe – A genetics testing service that uses genotyping to provide reports to individuals at affordable rates using a saliva sample. Reports reveal whether the person is a carrier of genetic variants for diseases. 23andMe customers can consent to participate in research in which their data are used to help power the work done by 23andMe scientists or third-party researchers, potentially contributing to hundreds of studies that range from Parkinson's disease to lupus to asthma.

» Counsyl – A genetics testing service that uses genotyping to provide reports to individuals using a provider-ordered blood sample. Depending on the healthcare provider, individuals may receive an email when results are ready (which would allow them to immediately download their results) or may be asked to schedule an appointment with one of Counsyl's genetic counselors who can help customers understand the results and what they mean. A consultation with a board-certified genetics counselor is included with every Counsyl screen.

Consumer Support–Informational –Decision-Making

» Accolade – An on-demand personalized advocacy and population health solution for employers, health plans, and consumers. Accolade uses independent health navigators to help people make the best decisions about their healthcare and to connect them to the resources they need.

» Buoy Health – An online symptom and cure checker that uses an intelligent algorithm backed by medical data to diagnose patients. It allows users to easily check symptoms and understand the best options for care, eliminating the need for Google searches and guessing.

» Clear Health Costs – A website for patients to compare prices on common procedures and doctor visits in select cities, and to check Medicare payment rates for thousands of procedures nationwide.

» Fair Health – A nonprofit that uses billing data to help patients estimate and plan their medical and dental expenses.

» Guroo – A tool created by the nonprofit Health Care Cost Institute to connect patients with information on cost and quality of care.

» Healthcare Blue Book – A fair price tool that allows patients to shop for affordable, high-quality care in their area.

» MediBid – A healthcare bidding site designed to connect patients with surgeons and specialists.

» Opencare – An online and mobile app to enable consumers to find the right dentist and to bring them together using a streamlined appointment booking platform. This serves as a gateway to simplifying all interactions between patients and dentists, ultimately making healthcare more personable, approachable, and accessible.

» PicnicHealth – An online portal that provides secure access to a consumer's medical records, enabling easier medical record management and coordination of care.

Provider Training

» Costs of Care – A nonprofit dedicated to helping prepare medical providers to look out for patients' wallets by considering unintentional financial harm from medical decisions providers make as they address patients' clinical needs. Costs of Care is helping to transform American healthcare delivery by empowering patients and their caregivers to deflate medical bills. High-value medical decisions benefit individual patients and society at large, and Costs of Care sees an opportunity to return $100 billion to the American people by helping medical providers replace or reject services that eat into consumers' wallets without making us healthier.

» Osso VR – A virtual reality surgical training platform designed for providers of all skill levels. This product offers highly realistic, hand-based interactions in an immersive training environment containing cutting-edge procedures and devices. Osso VR's training is results-driven, allowing teams and individuals to objectively measure their performance through the company's proprietary analytics platform and dashboards. Osso VR is currently focused on solving training gaps for orthopedic and spine therapies but is also expanding into other specialties and procedures.

» VLIPPmed – A global virtual reality platform providing healthcare professionals and medical students with access to real-life immersive training content through an innovative 360-degree experience.

Comparison Research

» Castlight Health – An online healthcare transparency
company that allows consumers to see the cost and
quality of care for surgeries and other medical services
at different providers. The Castlight platform is
licensed through a business-to-business subscription
model, so only employees of companies that have
purchased subscriptions have access to it. However,
some insurance companies may provide their
commercial members with access to the platform's
core price transparency tool.

» DirectHealth.com – An online health insurance
comparison site that is an independent licensed
health insurance agency that can provide unprecedented access to health insurance information and
enrollment support for consumers. DirectHealth.
com manages relationships with licensed insurance
agents, enabling consumers to compare coverage
options and enroll in a plan that is right for them
via online or telephone channels, or directly in 2,700
Walmart stores.

Personal Health Tracking

» Ada Health – A personal health companion that
builds a detailed picture of the consumer's personal
health over time, providing users with a simple and
personalized understanding of what is happening
with their bodies.

Research and Development

» Calico – A research and development company whose mission is to harness advanced technologies to increase our understanding of the biology that controls life-span. Calico will use that knowledge to devise interventions that enable people to lead longer and healthier lives.

Financial Services

» VisitPay – An online financial engagement platform that simplifies the entire billing experience for both patients and health systems—providing greater transparency, choice, and control. VisitPay underwrites payment options for each consumer, presents a single monthly bill and EOB information at the visit level, links with the consumer's HSA account, and consolidates accounts for consumers.

Information Sharing

» CareZone – A website and mobile app to help families easily share important information with loved ones and caretakers who need it. Provides a secure online space to store and privately share information such as emergency contact numbers, social security numbers, important insurance documents, doctors' appointments, directions on administering medications to loved ones, and other functions. The company also offers productivity tools such as journaling, to-do lists, calendars, data storage, and broadcast—a feature that enables users to record and send messages in real time to up to 100 contacts simultaneously.

DISRUPTIVE ORGANIZATIONS OUTSIDE HEALTHCARE

Here we highlight some of the major nonhealthcare disruptive organizations that are changing the competitive landscape by overturning existing business models and boundaries and rendering existing value propositions obsolete.

Retail

» Alibaba – Is to China what Amazon is to the US, and then some. Alibaba provides consumer-to-consumer, business-to-consumer, and business-to-business sales services via web portals. They also offer electronic payment services, shopping search engines, and cloud computing services. They own and operate a diverse array of businesses around the world in numerous sectors. Like Amazon, Alibaba has brought unprecedented levels of selection, price transparency, and convenience to business-to-business as well as to consumer retail shopping.

Entertainment

» Netflix – A streaming service that allows consumers to watch a wide variety of TV shows, movies, documentaries, and more on internet-connected devices. Their initial business model focused on DVD rental by mail, but subsequently expanded to include streaming media. Netflix entered the content-production industry in 2012 and has greatly expanded the production of both film and television series since then. In 2016, Netflix released an estimated 126 original series or films, more than any other network or cable channel. Netflix more than any other company has redefined how people consume entertainment.

Transportation

» Didi Chuxing – A major Chinese ridesharing, artificial intelligence, and autonomous technology conglomerate. It provides services including taxi hailing, private car hailing, social ride sharing, DiDi Designated Driving, DiDi Bus, DiDi Test Drive, DiDi Car Sharing, DiDi Enterprise Solutions, DiDi Minibus, DiDi Luxe, bike and e-bike sharing, and food delivery to users in China via a smartphone. Even more so than Uber and Lyft in the US, Didi is significantly shaking up transportation in China.

» Lyft – A peer-to-peer ridesharing, taxicab, bicycle sharing, and innovator with respect to electric scooters and other methods of transportation. Lyft has partnered with hospital systems and insurers (who pay the bill) to help patients get to medical treatments and dialysis centers. Lyft has also promised to reduce the healthcare transportation gap—the millions of Americans who miss medical appointments because they lack transportation—by 50 percent.

» Uber – A peer-to-peer ridesharing, taxicab, food delivery, bicycle sharing, and transportation network company. With its app-based hire-car sharing service, Uber changed the landscape for hired driving and has its sights set even higher, on transportation in general. In 2015, the company established Uber's Advanced Technologies Center to develop self-driving cars. Uber is also pursuing Uber Freight, which matches freight shippers with truckers in a similar fashion to the matching of taxi passengers with drivers.

Together, these organizations are redefining transportation and will ultimately challenge the notion of automobile ownership.

Hospitality

» Airbnb – An online marketplace and hospitality service specializing in connecting homeowners to customers looking for short-term rentals. Airbnb allows people to lease or rent everything from holiday cottages, apartments, home stays, hostel beds, hotel rooms, luxury villas, and even tree houses. The company also facilitates experiences—like walking tours and beach yoga—near one's destination and enables consumers to make reservations at restaurants. With respect to healthcare, Airbnb promotes an Open Homes program that patients and their families can access through the Make-A-Wish Foundation. Through this program Airbnb hosts are able to offer their homes to people undergoing medical treatment for free.

» VRBO – Vacation Rental by Owner was the original online marketplace specializing in vacation rentals of all types: houses, apartments, condos, villas. VRBO has been a key player in vacation rentals, helping pave the way for home sharing services since the mid-1990s. With VRBO the owner must rent the entire dwelling, they cannot rent out a single room as owners can with Airbnb.

Neither of these companies owns any real estate or conducts tours; they are brokers who receive a percentage service fee for every booking. The brokered, online vacation rental marketplace pioneered by these organizations has given consumers more choice in lodging options, increased travel across all demographic groups, and provided an added source of income for homeowners.

Financial Services

» Ally – A 100 percent online bank holding company that provides a variety of financial services including online banking, automobile finance and vehicle insurance, corporate lending, mortgages, credit cards, and brokerage firm services. Ally offers an innovative digital experience, 24/7 customer service via phone or online chat (there will always be a human being to interact with), great rates, rewarding credit and lending products, and managed investment products for nearly every level of investor, with some of the industry's lowest fees.

» Brightside – An online platform designed to reduce financial stress as well as increase users' net income and quality of life. Brightside provides one place for people to turn for all their financial needs and provides dedicated real-time expert guidance to optimize financial behavior, decision support and personalized financial products that improve net income, as well as unbiased service without any kickbacks or ads from financial institutions.

» WeChat – A Chinese multipurpose messaging, social media, and mobile payment app. It has become one of the world's largest stand-alone mobile apps—with over 1 billion monthly active users and 902 million daily active users—and is known as China's "app for everything" and a "super app" because of its wide range of functions and platforms. In addition to its Facebook-like social media and social networking services, WeChat's success has been powered by the platform's mobile payment service, WeChat Pay, which assists with every aspect of a user's life—from shopping and hailing taxis, to organizing hospital appointments and ordering food deliveries. Now expanding beyond China to other countries, WeChat is exporting mobile payment to the world. Its immense scale will ensure WeChat has a dramatic impact on global finance as people replace cash with mobile payments, and as mobile payments supersede traditional credit and debit cards. Because WeChat allows local merchants to receive payments to their account within a shorter time frame and at a lower transaction cost than credit cards, WeChat could potentially usurp Visa, MasterCard, and American Express.

Education

» Coursera, edX, Udacity, and others – online learning platforms that offer courses, specializations, and degrees in a variety of subjects. In their push to democratize learning by making it transparent and accessible to anyone with internet access, massive open online courses (MOOCs) have the potential to significantly disrupt higher education around the world. As employers come to recognize MOOCs as viable alternatives to traditional baccalaureate and graduate degrees, students around the world will decide to forgo universities by taking MOOCs and saving tens of thousands of dollars. Nonprofit organizations such as the Bill & Melinda Gates Foundation are exploring the potential of offering MOOCs to low-income students. Currently, it is not possible to know where or how far MOOCs will take higher education, but they are most certainly here to stay.

Social Media

» Facebook – An online social media and social networking service that makes it easy for people to connect and share with family and friends, discover what's going on in the world, and share/express what matters to them. Despite its less than inspired handling of user privacy, the psychological effects it has on users, and the amount of fake news, hate speech, and depictions of violence prevalent on its services (all of which it is attempting to counteract), Facebook enables users to discover connections with people who have shared interests, understand those connections better by following them, and uncover interesting stories that may not otherwise have been discovered. With more than 2.2 billion monthly active users, Facebook's impact on the media, economy, politics, and social issues cannot be understated.

» Snapchat – A multimedia messaging app used globally to share pictures and messages for a short time before they become inaccessible. The app has evolved from originally focusing on person-to-person photo sharing to currently performing a range of different functions, including sending short videos, live video chatting, messaging, creating caricature-like Bitmoji avatars, and sharing photos and videos via a chronological "story" that's broadcast to all of one's followers. There's even a designated "Discovery" area within the app that is designed to showcase short-form content from major publishers. Another feature includes the ability to send money through an integration with Square Cash. Snapchat has become notable for representing a new, mobile-first direction for social media and places significant emphasis on users interacting with virtual stickers and augmented reality objects.

» WeChat – A Chinese multipurpose messaging, social media, and mobile payment app described as one of the top financial services disruptors. In addition to shaking up financial services with WeChat Pay, their social media platform is to China what Facebook and Skype are in the US. WeChat makes it easy for over 1 billion Chinese to connect and share with family and friends, discover what's going on in the world, and share/express what matters to them. In July 2018 WeChat struck a deal to provide WebMD's content to the more than 1 billion users of WeChat's social network. This early foray into healthcare is the harbinger of things to come for China's social media titan.

Marketing / Advertising

» Red Bull – Content marketing company focused less on promoting the popular energy drink than it is on creating a brand that embodies a distinct (extreme) lifestyle and audience. Red Bull has been leading the way in content marketing—a pull strategy that attracts customers by delivering information that is educational, entertaining, and engaging. It's about being available to consumers when they are looking for you and is much more successful than interruption-based techniques. Red Bull remains unsurpassed in their ability to grow, innovate, and adapt in a world of content.

Technology

» Samsung – A South Korean multinational conglomerate composed of affiliated businesses in food
processing, textiles, insurance, securities, retail, construction, shipbuilding, and electronics. Increasingly
globalized in its activities, Samsung Electronics is one
of the world's largest and most innovative information
technology companies, consumer electronics makers,
and chipmakers.

Shared Spaces

» WeWork – An American-based global network of
shared workspaces for entrepreneurs, freelancers,
start-ups, small businesses, and large enterprises.
WeWork's goal is to transform buildings into dynamic
environments for creativity, focus, and connection
as well as to humanize work. Regarding healthcare,
WeWork has pledged to create new collaboration hubs
that will provide spaces for health researchers, patients,
and advocates to get together to improve healthcare.

In a league by itself...

» Tencent Holdings Limited – A Chinese multinational
investment holding conglomerate whose subsidiaries
specialize in various internet-related services and
products, entertainment, artificial intelligence, and
technology, both in China and globally. Tencent
created WeChat and is one of the world's biggest
investment corporations, one of the largest internet
and technology companies, one of the biggest ven-
ture capital firms, and the largest and most valuable
gaming and social media company.

ENDNOTES

Preface: Healthcare Is Killing US—Physically, Financially, and Spiritually

1. Martin Makary and Michael Daniel, "Study Suggests Medical Errors Now Third Leading Cause of Death in the U.S.," *BMJ*, May 3, 2016.

2. Melonie Heron, "Deaths: Leading Causes for 2016," *National Vital Statistics Report*, Volume 67, Number 6, July 26, 2018.

3. Sophia Bernazzani, "Tallying the High Cost of Preventable Harm," Costs of Care, October 5, 2016.

4. Anna Medaris Miller, "5 Common Preventable Medical Errors and What You Can Do to Protect Yourself Against Them," *U.S. News and World Report* Online, March 30, 2015.

5. David C. Classen, Roger Resar, Frances Griffin, Frank Federico, Terri Frankel, Nancy Kimmel, John C. Whittington, Allan Frankel, Andrew Seger, and Brent C. James, "Global Trigger Tool Shows That Adverse Events in Hospitals May Be Ten Times Greater Than Previously Measured," *Health Affairs*, April 2011.

6. Jill Van Den Bos, Karan Rustagi, Travis Gray, Michael Halford, Eva Ziemkiewicz, and Jonathan Shreve, "The $17.1 Billion Problem: The Annual Cost of Measurable Medical Errors," *Health Affairs*, April 2011.

7. Jon Shreve, Jill Van Den Bos, Travis Gray, Michael Halford, Karan Rustagi, and Eva Ziemkiewicz, "The Economic Measurement of Medical Errors," The Society of Actuaries, June 2010.

8. National Institute on Drug Abuse, "Overdose Death Rates," revised January 2019.

9. Dave Chase, "The Opioid Crisis Wake-Up Call," Health Rosetta Media, September 4, 2018.

10. "10 Statistics about US Medical Debt That Will Shock You," National Bankruptcy Forum, December 14, 2017.

11. Leslie Kane, "National Physician Burnout, Depression & Suicide Report 2019," Medscape, January 16, 2019.

Introduction

1. Gigi A. Cuckler, Andrea M. Sisko, John A. Poisal, Sean P. Keehan, Sheila D. Smith, Andrew J. Madison, Christian J. Wolfe, and James C. Hardesty, "National Health Expenditure Projections, 2017–26: Despite Uncertainty, Fundamentals Primarily Drive Spending Growth," *Health Affairs*, February 14, 2018.

2. Megan Beck and Barry Libert, "Three Signals Your Industry Is about to Be Disrupted," *MIT Sloan Management* Review, June 11, 2018.

3. Sean Wise, "These 3 Industries Are Ready to Be Disrupted, Are You Going to Be the One to Do It?" *Inc*, July 12, 2018.

4. Melanie Evans, "Amazon Makes Inroads Selling Medical Supplies to the Sick," *Wall Street Journal*, November 29, 2018.

5. Jessica Kim Cohen, "Google Turns 20: Here Are 7 Ways It's Changing Healthcare," *Becker's Health IT & CIO Report*, September 10, 2018.

6. Scott Van Voorhis, "Microsoft Shares Up after Major Health Care Deal with Walgreens," *The Street*, January 15, 2019.

7. Paul Leinwant and Cesare Mainardi, "The Fear of Disruption Can Be More Damaging than Actual Disruption," *Strategy+Business*, September 27, 2017.

8. Jennifer Reynolds, "Travel Trends by Age Demographic."

9. "Disruptors and the Disrupted: A Tale of Eight Companies—In Pictures," *Strategy+Business Tech & Innovation*, September 27, 2017.

Chapter 1 – Why the Band-Aid Is about to Be Ripped off Traditional Healthcare

1. Ken Dychtwald, *Age Wave: How the Most Important Trend of Our Time Will Change Your Future*, Bantam Books, February 1990.

2. Ken Dychtwald, "Will the Age Wave Make or Break America? The Questions That Trump, Clinton and Sanders Must Answer," *Huffington Post*, May 5, 2016, updated May 19, 2017.

3. Caroline Humer, "Fed Up with Rising Costs, Big U.S. Firms Dig into Healthcare," Reuters, June 11, 2018.

4. Christina Farr and Lauren Hirsch, "Amazon Could Do a Lot to Fix the U.S. Health-care System—but Walmart Could Do More," CNBC, April 4, 2018.

5. Jed Graham, "Walmart, Not Amazon, May Turn Out to Be the Real Health Care Disruptor," *Investor's Business Daily*, April 2, 2018.

6. Steven Porter, "When Retail Giants Like Walmart and Amazon Invade Healthcare," *HealthLeaders*, June 18, 2018.

7. Tami Luhby, "Walmart Wants to Bring Its 'Everyday Low Prices' to Health Care," CNN Money, September 19, 2018.

8. Nathaniel Meyersohn and Tami Luhby, "Why Walmart May Want to Buy Humana," CNN Money, March 30, 2018.

9. Corporate Walmart, Company Facts.

10. Reed Abelson, "The Last Company You Would Expect Is Reinventing Health Benefits," *New York Times*, August 31, 2018.

11. Daniel Frankel, "Employee Headcount: The Rise and Fall of Job Numbers at Comcast, Charter, Altice and More," FierceVideo, a division of Questex, July 19, 2017.

12. Anna Wilde Mathews, "GM Cuts Different Type of Health-Care Deal," *Wall Street Journal*, August 6, 2018.

13. Ana Gupta and Daniel Grosslight, "Payor Services/A Call to Action: Can Large Employers Disintermediate the Big 4 MCO?" Leerink, October 5, 2018.

14. Caroline Humer, "Fed Up with Rising Costs, Big U.S. Firms Dig into Healthcare," Reuters, June 11, 2018.

15. Naseem S. Miller, "Disney Partnering with Orlando Health, Florida Hospital to Offer HMO Plans," *Orlando Sentinel,* February, 21, 2019.

16. Ayla Ellison, "Boeing, Cisco, Intel and Walmart Are Bypassing Insurers to Drive Down Healthcare Costs," *Becker's Healthcare Hospital CFO Report,* June 11, 2018.

17. Keith Speights, "Forget Obamacare and Trumpcare: Boeing, GE, and Other Companies Are Reforming Healthcare on Their Own," The Motley Fool, June 25, 2017.

18. Corey Noles, "Boeing Taps into Mercy Health Insurance Offering," *St. Louis Business Journal,* July 31, 2015.

19. Stephen E. Littlejohn, "Boeing, Going, Gone: The End of Group Health Insurance," *Pharmaceutical Executive,* August 4, 2015.

20. Jonathan R. Slotkin, Olivia A. Ross, M. Ruth Coleman, and Jaewon Ryu, "Why GE, Boeing, Lowe's, and Walmart Are Directly Buying Health Care for Employees," *Harvard Business Review,* June 8, 2017.

21. Pacific Business Group on Health, "Employers Centers of Excellence Network."

22. "Some Hospital Emergency Department Visits Could Be Handled by Alternative Care Settings," RAND Corporation, September 7, 2010 (News Release).

23. Doug Pfaff, "The Emergence of Choice: Why Consumers Own the Future of Healthcare," Huron.

24. Vijay Govindarajan and Ravi Ramamurti, "Transforming Healthcare from the Ground Up," *Harvard Business Review,* July–August 2018, pp. 96–104.

25. "Excerpt from Outpatient Surgical Centers Industry Profile," Outpatient Surgical Centers Industry Profile, Dun & Bradstreet First Research, December, 3, 2018.

26. Kaiser Health News, "Readers Seek Transparency on Surgery Centers 'Bill of the Month' Investigations," *Washington Post,* March 28, 2018.

27. Christina Jewett and Mark Alesia, "As Surgery Centers Boom, Patients Are Paying with Their Lives," Kaiser Health New, March 2, 2018.

28. Christina Jewett and Mark Alesia, "How a Push to Cut Costs and Boost Profits at Surgery Centers Led to a Trail of Death," *USA TODAY,* March 5, 2018.

29. "Will Ambulatory Surgery Centers Become More 'Hospital-Like'?" SSI.

30. Free Market Medical Association.

31. The founders of FMMA have approved our inclusion of information about FMMA as well as the inclusion of their pillars.

32. Joyce Friedan, "A Big Medical Tourism Boom? Actually, Not So Much—The Industry Hasn't Worked out as Its Supporters Expected," MedPage Today, May 2, 2018.

33. Robert Pearl, "U.S. Health Care Needs a Wake-up Call from India: Column," *USA TODAY,* January 29, 2017.

34. Cyber Knife Center, Cancer Clinic, Hamburg, Germany.

35. "International Hospital Management Corporation Chooses Allscripts Sunrise," Allscripts, (Globe Newswire), February 11, 2015.

36. "Healthcare in the United Arab Emirates," Wikipedia.

37. "Our History–Dubai Health Authority," Archived 2013-03-24 at the Wayback Machine.

38. "Medical Tourism Market Worth $179.6 Billion by 2026 CAGR: 21.9%," Grand View Research, February 2019.

39. "Compare Prices," Medical Tourism, 2019.

40. "Medical Procedure Cost Comparison by Country," Brokerfish.

41. Vijay Govindarajan and Ravi Ramamurti, "Is This the Hospital That Will Finally Push the Expensive U.S. Health Care System to Innovate?" *Harvard Business Review*, June 22, 2018.

42. Bertalan Mesko, "12 Things We Can 3D Print in Medicine Right Now," 3D Printing Industry, February 26, 2015.

43. "Medical Applications of 3D Printing," US Food and Drug Administration, December 4, 2017.

44. Nancy S. Giges, "Top 5 Ways 3D Printing Is Changing the Medical Field," ASME, May 2017.

45. "Healthcare Innovation Map Reveals Emerging Technologies & Startups," StartUs Insights.

46. InnovationOchsner Brochure.

47. "Healthcare Innovation Map Reveals Emerging Technologies & Startups," StartUs Insights.

48. "Using AI to meet operational, clinical goals," *Becker's Healthcare, Becker's Hospital Review.*

49. Marco Iansiti and Karim R. Lakhani, "The Truth about Blockchain," *Harvard Business Review*, January–February 2017, pp. 118–27.

50. "How Blockchain Technology Could Disrupt Healthcare," CB Insights Research Report.

51. Kate Rooney, "Despite Cryptocurrency Crash, Amazon Sees Opportunity to Embrace Blockchain," CNBC, November 29, 2018.

52. Andrew Twite, "Electric Vehicles: Good for Public Health and the Planet," Fresh Energy, June 20, 2017.

53. Jennifer Chu, "Study: Air Pollution Causes 200,000 Early Deaths Each Year in the U.S.," MIT News, August 29, 2013.

Chapter 2 – A Disruptive Antidote: Curing Our Ailing System in a Life or Death World

1. Mathias Herzog, Tom Puthiyamadam, and Nils Naujok, "10 Principles for Winning the Game of Digital Disruption," *Strategy+Business, Tech & Innovation*, November 30, 2017.

2. Brooke Murphy, "8 of the Most Memorable Quotes about Hospital Prices," *Becker's Healthcare, Hospital CFO Report*, August 24, 2016.

3. David Edelburg, "The Insanity of Healthcare Pricing," Whole Health Chicago.

4. Sarah Kliff, "The Absurdity of American Health Care Pricing, in One Chart," Vox, May 9, 2018.

5. Sarah Kliff, "These 15 Charts Show Our Health Care Prices Are Totally Insane," Vox, May 31, 2015.

6. Jaime A Rosenthal, Xin Lu, and Peter Cram, "Availability of Consumer Prices from US Hospitals for a Common Surgical Procedure," JAMA Network, *JAMA Internal Medicine*, March 25, 2013.

7. Jeffrey Young and Chris Kirkham, "Hospital Prices No Longer Secret as New Data Reveals Bewildering System, Staggering Cost Differences," *Huffington Post*, May 8, 2013, updated December 6, 2017.

8. David E. Williams, "The Insanity of Health Care Pricing, aka Alice in Medical Land," Health Care Blog, March 1, 2011.

9. Chad Terhune, "His $109K Heart Attack Bill Is Now Down to $332 after NPR Told His Story," NPR, *All Things Considered*, August 31, 2018.

10. Sarah Kliff, "The Problem Is the Prices—Opaque and Sky High Bills Are Breaking Americans—and Our Health Care System." Vox, October 16, 2017.

11. Fred Schulte, "Pain Hits after Surgery When a Doctor's Daughter Is Stunned by $17,850 Urine Test," Kaiser Health News, February 16, 2018.

12. Evette Dion, "One Man's Ridiculous Hospital Bill Sums up the Problem with America's Healthcare," Revelist, November 3, 2016.

13. Sarah Kliff, "She Didn't Get Treated at the ER. But She Got a $5,751 Bill Anyway," Vox, May 1, 2018.

14. Sarah Kliff, "The Case of the $629 Band-Aid—and What It Reveals about American Health Care," Vox, May 13, 2016.

15. R. Scott Munro, "37 Quotes on Health Care and Health Tech from 2016," Medium, January 2, 2017.

16. Scott Atlas, "The Path to Affordable Health Care," Hoover Institution, Defining Ideas, November 30, 2017.

17. Melanie Evans, "What Does Knee Surgery Cost? Few Know, and That's a Problem," *Wall Street Journal*, August 21, 2018.

18. Brooke Murphy, "8 of the Most Memorable Quotes about Hospital Prices," *Becker's Healthcare, Hospital CFO Report*, August 24, 2016.

19. "Medicare Provider Utilization and Payment Data," CMS.gov, August 10, 2017.

20. Sarah Kliff, "How Much Does an Appendectomy Cost? Somewhere between $1,529 and $186,955," *Washington Post*, April 24, 2012.

21. Sarah Kliff and Dan Keating, "One Hospital Charges $800—Another, $38,000," *Washington Post*, May 8, 2013.

22. Bob Herman, "The Striking Variation of Commercial Healthcare Prices," *Modern Healthcare*, April 27, 2016.

23. Sarah Kliff, "The Absurdity of American Health Care Pricing, in One Chart," Vox, May 9, 2018.

24. Jayne O'Donnell, "Huge Healthcare Price Differences Even within Same Area, by State," *USA TODAY*, April 27, 2016, updated April 29, 2016.

25. Luca Dezzani, "Healthcare Costs in the World," Igea Hub Pharmaceutical Club, February 5, 2017.

26. Rabah Kamal and Cynthia Cox, "How Do Healthcare Prices and Use in the U.S. Compare to Other Countries?" Peterson-Kaiser Health System Tracker, May 8, 2018.

27. Jeff Byers, "iFHP Cost Report Highlights Cause for Concern over Lack of Provider Competition," Healthcare Dive, July 19, 2016.

28. Lee Beecher with David Racer, *Passion for Patients*, Alethos Press (Bloomington, MN: Bethany Press International), 2017.

29. "The Case for Transparency: Why It Pays to Empower Patient Choice," Parallon Study.

30. Lisa Schencker, "Why Don't More People Shop for Health Care? Online Tools Exist, but Most Don't Use Them," *Chicago Tribune*, July 20, 2018.

31. Jessica Silver-Greenberg, "How to Fight a Bogus Bill," *Wall Street Journal*, February 19, 2011.

32. Sarah Kliff, "A Woman Had a Baby. Then Her Hospital Charged Her $39.35 to Hold It," Vox, October 4, 2016.

33. Tamara Rosin and Emily Rappleye, "On the Record: 50 Best Healthcare Quotes of 2016," *Becker's Healthcare, Hospital Review*, December 27, 2016.

34. Jennie Situ, "Addressing Transportation Issues Leads to Better Care," Hospitals & Health Networks, December 7, 2017.

35. Samina T. Syed, Ben S. Gerber, and Lisa K. Sharp, "Traveling Towards Disease: Transportation Barriers to Health Care Access," NCBI Resources, PMC, US National Library of Medicine, National Institute of Health, *J Community Health*, October, 2013.

36. Parija Kavilanz, "The US Can't Keep up with Demand for Health Aides, Nurses and Doctors," CNN Money, May 4, 2018.

37. Megan Knowles, "Rural North Carolina Hospital Uses Walmart Clinic to Ease Pressure on ED," *Becker's Healthcare, Becker's Hospital Review*, September 10, 2018.

38. William W. Chin, Richard G. Hamermesh, Robert S. Huckman, Barbara J. McNeil, and Joseph P. Newhouse, "5 Imperatives Addressing Healthcare's Innovation Challenge," Harvard Business School, Harvard Medical School, Forum on Healthcare Innovation, 2012.

39. Vijay Govindarajan and Ravi Ramamurti, "Transforming Healthcare from the Ground Up," *Harvard Business Review*, July–August 2018, pp. 96–104.

40. "Healthcare Innovation Map Reveals Emerging Technologies & Startups," StartUs Insights.

41. James A. Bacon, "The Future of Health Care Delivery: Homes Not Hospitals," Bacon's Rebellion, February 26, 2018.

42. Erin M. Kelly, "The History of Physician House Calls," MultiCare House Call Physicians, June 29, 2017.

43. "The Test Drive That Comes to You," Hyundai USA website.

44. Thomas M. Maddux, BJC Innovation Lab Strategic Plan, Barnes Jewish Hospital, St. Louis, MO.

45. Scott Atlas, "The Path to Affordable Health Care," Hoover Institution, Defining Ideas, November 30, 2017.

46. "New MGMA Data Shows Medical Practices Utilizing More Non-Physician Providers Are More Profitable, Productive," Medical Group Management Association Press Release, 2018.

47. "New Research Shows Increasing Physician Shortages in Both Primary and Specialty Care," Association of American Medical Colleges Press Release, April 11, 2018.

48. Pam Koenig, "Chronic Disease as a Result of Poor Lifestyle Choices," Eastport Health Care, Inc., October 10, 2014.

49. "Measuring the Risks and Causes of Premature Death: Summary of Workshops," National Research Council and Institute of Medicine, Washington, DC, 2015.

50. "Become a Health Coach," Health Coach Institute.

51. David Epstein and Propublica, "When Evidence Says No, but Doctors Say Yes," *Atlantic*, February 22, 2017.

52. Atul Gawande, "Overkill, An Avalanche of Unnecessary Medical Care Is Harming Patients Physically and Financially. What Can We Do about It?" *New Yorker, Annals of Health Care*, May 11, 2015.

53. Mark S. Klempner, Linden T. Hu, Janine Evans, Christopher H. Schmid, Gary M. Johnson, Richard P. Trevino, DeLona Norton, Lois Levy, Dian Wall, John McCall, Mark Kosinski, and Arthur Weinstein, "Two Controlled Trials of Antibiotic Treatment in Patients with Persistent Symptoms and a History of Lyme Disease," *New England Journal of Medicine*, July 12, 2001.

54. Elliot Bennett-Guerrero, Theodore N. Pappas, Walter A. Koltun, James W. Fleshman, Min Lin, Jyotsna Garg, Daniel B. Mark, Jorge E. Marcet, Feza H. Remzi, Virgilio V. George, Kerstin Newland, and G. R. Corey, for the SWIPE 2 Trial Group, "Gentamicin—Collagen Sponge for Infection Prophylaxis in Colorectal Surgery," *New England Journal of Medicine*, September 9, 2010.

55. Adam G. Elshaug, Amber M. Watt, Linda Mundy, and Cameron D. Willis, "Over 150 Potentially Low-value Health Care Practices: an Australian Study," *Medical Journal of Australia*, Volume 197, Issue 10, November 19, 2012.

56. Vinay Prasad, Andrae Vandross, Caitlin Toomey, Michael Cheung, Jason Rho, Steven Quinn, Satish Jacob Chacko, Durga Borkar, Victor Gail, Senthil Selvaraj, Nancy Ho, and Adam Cifu, "A Decade of Reversal: An Analysis of 146 Contradicted Medical Practices," *Mayo Clinic Proceedings*, August 2013, Volume 88, Issue 8, pp. 790–798.

57. John P. A. Ioannidis, "Editorial: How Many Contemporary Medical Practices Are Worse Than Doing Nothing or Doing Less?" *Mayo Clinic Proceedings*, August 2013, Volume 88, Issue 8, pp. 779–781.

58. Anthony Sagel, "How 6 Months with Florence, My Virtual Assistant, Helped Me and My Patients," Nuance, Healthcare, March 29, 2017.

59. Priyanka Dayal McCluskey, "Meet Eva, the Voice-activated 'Assistant' for Doctors," *Boston Globe*, January 9, 2018.

60. David Marino-Nachison, "Digital Assistants: Why Your Doctor Should Talk to Alexa," *Barron's*, February 12, 2018.

61. Pam Baker, "The Robot Will See You Now," Hewlett Packard Enterprise, enterprise.nxt, August 2, 2017.

62. "It's Early Days for the Use of AI in Medicine," *Wall Street Journal*, Opinion, August 13, 2018.

63. Danielle Sabrina, "How the Membership Business Model Is Changing the Way We Buy," *Huffington Post*, July 11, 2016.

64. Shep Hyken, "How to Create a Membership Model and Boost Your Business," *Forbes*, July 23, 2015.

65. Will Ford, "Why the Membership Model Makes Sense," *Entrepreneur*, April 8, 2015.

66. Les Masterson, "Louisiana Launching 'Netflix Model' in Medicaid for Hepatitis C Drugs," Healthcare Dive, January 14, 2019.

67. Carol Y. Johnson, "Louisiana Adopts 'Netflix' Model to Pay for Hepatitis C Drugs," *Washington Post*, January 10, 2019.

68. Lydia Ramsey, "A New Kind of Doctor's Office Charges a Monthly Fee and Doesn't Take Insurance—and It Could Be the Future of Medicine," *Business Insider*, March 19, 2017.

69. Steve Jacob, "Why Concierge Medicine Is Good for Patients—and Physicians," *D Magazine* Special Report, Dallas Medical Directory, 2012.

70. Planetree International. The Official Website of Planetree International.

71. Ellen Wehle, "7 Things I Learned from Atul Gawande's *Being Mortal*," Barnes & Noble News Releases, October 6, 2014.

72. Todd Ferguson, "Creating Healing Environments with Evidence-Based Design," OH&S, October 1, 2010.

73. America's Health Rankings, United Health Foundation, 2018.

74. "Cleveland Clinic Study Finds Obesity as Top Cause of Preventable Life-Years Lost," Newsroom, Cleveland Clinic News Release, April 22, 2017.

75. Holly Brenza, "Move Over, Tobacco—There's a New Leading Cause of Preventable Death," health enews, Advocate Aurora Health, Advocate Medical Group.

76. "Adult Obesity Facts—Obesity Is Common, Serious, and Costly," Centers for Disease Control and Prevention, August 13, 2018.

77. Su-Hsin Chang, Lisa M. Pollack, and Graham A. Colditz, "Life Years Lost Associated with Obesity-Related Diseases for U.S. Non-Smoking Adults," *PLOS ONE*, NCBI, PMC, US National Library of Medicine, National Institutes of Health, June 18, 2013.

78. Alan Kohll, "8 Things You Need to Know about Employee Wellness Programs," *Forbes*, April 21, 2016.

79. Nancy S. Mure, *Eat! Empower. Adjust. Triumph!* YourSpecs, an imprint of SynergEbooks, 2015.

80. Employee Financial Wellness Program, GreenPath financial wellness.

81. Stephen Miller, "Employee's Financial Issues Affect Their Job Performance," SHRM, April 29, 2016.

82. "8 Megatrends Driving Disruption," Ernst & Young Brochure.

83. "Measuring the Risks and Causes of Premature Death: Summary of Workshops," National Research Council and Institute of Medicine, Washington, DC, 2015.

84. Thomas M. Maddux, BJC Innovation Lab Strategic Plan. Barnes Jewish Hospital, St. Louis, MO, 2018.

85. "How to Build Healthy Communities," Plan H, BC Healthy Communities Society, British Columbia, Canada.

86. "Building Healthy Communities Program," Blue Cross Blue Shield of Michigan.

87. "Building Healthy Communities Fact Sheet," Blue Cross Blue Shield of Michigan.

88. "Building Healthy Communities," Official Website of the City of New York.

89. "Building a Healthy Community Together," Johns Hopkins Medicine Website.

CHAPTER 3 – HOW HEALTHCARE CAN MEDICATE ITSELF: A BIG, BITTERSWEET DOSE OF DISRUPTION

1. Karim Benammar, "Reframing/The Art of Thinking Differently," Uitgeverij Boom, Amsterdam, 2012.

2. Yasmeen Abutaleb, "FDA's Gottlieb Blames Industry 'Kabuki Drug Pricing' for High Costs," Reuters, March 7, 2018.

3. Heather Fernandez, "The Rise of the Practical Patient: What Do Healthcare Consumers Really Want?" Solv, May 1, 2018.

4. "Rise of the Practical Patient," Solv Consumer Healthcare Report, 2018.

5. Robert B. Tucker, "How Does Amazon Do It? Five Critical Factors That Explain Amazon's Incredible Success," *Forbes*, November 1, 2018.

6. Chris Weber, "Introducing Uber Health, Removing Transportation as a Barrier to Care," Uber Newsroom, March 1, 2018.

7. Jennifer Surane and Christopher Cannon, "Why China's Payment Apps Give U.S. Bankers Nightmares," Bloomberg, May 23, 2018.

8. Vijay Govindarajan and Ravi Ramamurti, "Transforming Healthcare from the Ground Up," *Harvard Business Review,* July–August, 2018, pp. 96–104.

9. Clayton Christensen, Karen Dillon, David Duncan, and Taddy Hall, "5 Ways to Identify the Best Innovation Opportunities," *Inc.*, October 2016.

CHAPTER 4 – FROM SICK CARE TO HEALTHCARE: WHO GETS HARMED, WHO GETS HELPED, AND WHO GETS IN THE WAY

1. "Hospital Errors Are the Third Leading Cause of Death in U.S., and New Hospital Safety Scores Show Improvements Are Too Slow," Leapfrog Hospital Safety Grade, October 23, 2013.

2. Kenneth E. Covinsky, Edgar Pierluissi, and C. Bree Johnston, "Hospitalization-Associated Disability, 'She Was Probably Able to Ambulate, but I'm Not Sure,'" *JAMA*, October 26, 2011.

3. Anna Gorman, "The Older You Are, the Worse the Hospital Is for You," CNN Health Online, August 15, 2016.

4. "Why Elderly Patients Often Leave the Hospital More Disabled Than When They Arrived," Advisory Board, August 15, 2016.

5. Marcia Angell, "A Better Way Out," *New York Review of Books*, January 8, 2015.

6. "Per-capita End-of-life Spending Is Decreasing Rapidly, According to New Study," Science Daily, The Dartmouth Institute for Health Policy & Clinical Practice, May 16, 2018.

7. Melissa D. Aldridge and Amy S. Kelley, "The Myth Regarding the High Cost of End-of-Life Care," NCBI, PMC, US National Library of Medicine, National Institutes of Health, *American Journal of Public Health,* December 2015.

8. Eric B. French et al., "End-of-Life Medical Spending in Last Twelve Months of Life Is Lower Than Previously Reported," *Health Affairs*, Vol. 36, No. 7, July 2017.

9. Sandra Levy, "End-of-Life Care: What Doctors Want for Themselves Differs from What They Provide Patients," *Healthline*, June 3, 2014.

10. "Death with Dignity Acts," Death with Dignity National Center.

11. Anna Gorman, "Hospitals Rethink Care for Elderly in Wake of Poor Outcomes," MedCity News, August 10, 2016.

12. Deborah E. Barnes, Robert M. Palmer, Denise M. Kresevic, Richard H. Fortinsky, Jerome Kowal, Mary-Margaret Chren, and C. Seth Landefeld, "Acute Care for Elders Units Produced Shorter Hospital Stays at Lower Cost While Maintaining Patients' Functional Status," *Health Affairs*, Vol. 31, No. 6, June 2012.

13. John Henley, "At My Father's Bedside, I Learned What Death Looks Like," *The Guardian*, February 3, 2016.

14. Anne Tumlinson, "The 5 Most Unexpected Challenges of Caregiving," *Huffington Post*, October 1, 2015, updated September 30, 2016.

15. "Challenges Facing Family Caregivers," Concordia, December 19, 2016.

16. "Does Our Future Depend on Elder Care Robots?" Waypoint Robotics Website.

17. Michelle Seitzer, "Top Tech Devices That Help Seniors Live at Home Comfortably and Safely," Care.com Community, September 12, 2018.

18. Laurie Beaver, "Big Tech in Healthcare: How Alphabet, Amazon, Apple, and Microsoft Are Shaking up Healthcare—and What It Means for the Future of the Industry," *Business Insider*, July 19, 2018.

19. Tim Regan, "Home Health Care Makes Inroads with Amazon Alexa Pilot," *Home Health Care News*, August 10, 2017.

20. Libby Kielb, "Libertana Home Health Deploys Orbita Voice Experience Software to Provide Amazon Echo-Based Digital Care Assistants in Community-Based Housing Environments," *Orbita*, August 10, 2017.

21. Eric Wicklund, "How One Home Health Provider Turned Alexa into an mHealth Assistant," mHealth Intelligence, xtelligent Healthcare Media, February 26, 2018.

22. Imani Moise, "For the Elderly Who Are Lonely, Robots Offer Companionship," *Wall Street Journal*, May 28, 2018.

23. Andrew Tarantola, "Robot Caregivers Are Saving the Elderly from Lives of Loneliness," Engadget, August 29, 2017.

24. "Importance of Good Nutrition" and "The Impact of Nutrition on Your Health," HHS.gov, President's Council on Sports, Fitness & Nutrition.

25. Data, Trends and Maps Database, Centers for Disease Control and Prevention, December 4, 2018.

26. "Measuring the Risks and Causes of Premature Death: Summary of Workshops," National Research Council and Institute of Medicine, Washington, DC, 2015.

27. Robyn Burton and Nick Sheron, "No Level of Alcohol Consumption Improves Health," *Lancet*, Vol. 392, Issue 10152, pp. 987–88, September 22, 2018.

28. Dirk De Ridder, Patrick Manning, Sook Ling Leong, Samantha Ross, Wayne Sutherland, Caroline Horwath, and Sven Vanneste, "The Brain, Obesity and Addiction: An EEG Neuroimaging Study," Scientific Reports, Scientific Reports 6, Article number: 34122(2016) September, 2016.

29. Amy Reichelt, "Fact or Fiction—Is Sugar Addictive," The Conversation, February 22, 2017.

30. Eric Bowman, "Explainer: What Is Dopamine—and Is It to Blame for Our Addictions?" The Conversation, December 3, 2015.

31. Joseph Nordqvist, "How Much Sugar Is in Your Food and Drink?" Medical News Today, February 14, 2018.

32. Jillian Kubala, "11 Reasons Why Too Much Sugar Is Bad for You," Healthline, June 3, 2018.

33. Sara F. L. Kirk and Jessie-Lee McIsaac, "Is the Food Industry Conspiring to Make You Fat?" The Conversation, August 9, 2017.

34. "Making the World Safe from Superbugs," *Consumer Reports*, Special Report, America's Antibiotic Crisis, November 18, 2015.

35. Maryn McKenna, "The Hidden Link Between Farm Antibiotics and Human Illness," *Wired*, September 7, 2018.

36. "2016 Summary Report on Antimicrobials Sold or Distributed for Use in Food-Producing Animals," US Food & Drug Administration, December 2017.

37. "Antibiotic/Antimicrobial Resistance (AR/AMR)," Centers for Disease Control and Prevention, September 10, 2018.

38. Christian Lindmeier, "Stop Using Antibiotics in Healthy Animals to Prevent the Spread of Antibiotic Resistance," World Health Organization, News Release, November 7, 2017.

39. Brian Owens, "Strategies to Reduce the Use of Antibiotics in Animals," *Pharmaceutical Journal*, November 11, 2014.

40. Tami Luhby, "The Real Story of Food Stamps," CNN Money, CNN Business, February 13, 2018.

41. Moby, "Food Stamps Shouldn't Pay for Junk," *Wall Street Journal*, April 9, 2018.

42. James Rettig, "Moby Pens WSJ Op-Ed Arguing That Food Stamps Shouldn't Pay for Junk Food," *Billboard*, April 11, 2018.

43. Rebecca L. Franckle et al., "Transactions at a Northeastern Supermarket Chain: Differences by Supplemental Nutrition Assistance Program Use," *American Journal of Preventive Medicine*, Vol. 53, Issue 4, pp. 131–138, October 2017.

44. "Diet Quality of Americans by SNAP Participation Status: Data from the National Health and Nutrition Examination Survey, 2007–2010—Summary," US Department of Agriculture, Food and Nutrition Service, May 2015.

45. Alisha Coleman-Jensen, Christian A. Gregory, and Matthew P. Rabbitt, "Measurement." US Department of Agriculture, Economic Research Service, August 20, 2018.

46. Alisha Coleman-Jensen, Christian A. Gregory, and Matthew P. Rabbitt, "Key Statistics & Graphics," US Department of Agriculture, Economic Research Service, September 5, 2018.

47. Nancy Weinfield, Gregory Mills, Christine Borger, Maeve Gearning, Theodore Macaluso, Jill Montaquila, and Sheila Zedlewski, "Hunger in America 2014: National Report Prepared for Feeding America," Westat and Urban Institute, August 2014.

48. Kostas Stamoulis, "FAO's Strategic Objective 1: Help Eliminate Hunger, Food Insecurity and Malnutrition," Food and Agriculture Organization of the United Nations, 2015.

49. J.B. Cordaro, "New Business Models to Help Eliminate Food and Nutrition INsecurity: Roadmap for Exploration," Paper presented at the ICN2 Second International Conference on Nutrition, November 19–21, 2014, Rome, Italy.

50. Ketaki Gokhale, "The Same Pill That Costs $1,000 in the U.S. Sells for $4 in India." *Chicago Tribune*, January 4, 2016

51. Beth Mole, "Years after Mylan's Epic EpiPen Price Hikes, It Finally Gets a Generic Rival," arsTECHNICA, August 17, 2018.

52. Matthew Herper, "The Cost of Creating a New Drug Now $5 Billion, Pushing Big Pharma to Change," *Forbes*, August 11, 2013.

53. Jessica Wapner, "How Prescription Drugs Get Their Prices, Explained," *Newsweek*, March 17, 2017.

54. Wayne Winegarden, "The Bizarre World of Drug Pricing," *Forbes*, November 19, 2018.

55. Charles Sliver and David A. Hyman, "Here's a Plan to Fight High Drug Prices That Could Unite Libertarians and Socialists," Vox, June 21, 2018.

56. Kate Bachelder Odell, "When Medical Innovation Meets Politics," *Wall Street Journal*, August 24, 2018.

57. Alia Paavola, "400% Price Hike for Generic Drug a 'Moral Requirement,' Missouri Pharma CEO says," *Becker's Healthcare, Becker's Hospital Review*, September 11, 2018.

58. Andrew Pollack, "Drug Goes from $13.50 a Tablet to $750, Overnight," *New York Times*, September 20, 2015.

59. Wayne Drash, "Anatomy of a 97,000% drug price hike: One Family's Fight to Save Their Son," CNN Health, June 29, 2018.

60. Sarah Kliff, "The True Story of America's Sky-high Prescription Drug Prices," Vox, May 10, 2018.

61. Henry I. Miller, "Follow the FDA's Self-Interest," *Wall Street Journal*, October 28, 2018.

62. Luca Dezzani, "Health Care Costs in the World," IGEA Hub Pharmaceutical Club, February 5, 2017.

63. Ben Hirschler, "How the U.S. Pays 3 Times More for Drugs," *Scientific American*, Reuters.

64. Anupam B. Jena, "US Drug Prices Higher Than in the Rest of the World, Here's Why," The Hill, January 19, 2018.

65. Robin Feldman, "May Your Drug Price be Evergreen," Journal of Law and the Biosciences, December 7, 2018.

66. The Editorial Board, "Why Are Drugs Cheaper in Europe?" *Wall Street Journal*, October 28, 2018.

67. Evan Sweeney, "Class-action Suit Claims Express Scripts Charges 'Exorbitant and Unlawful' Medical Records Fees," Fierce Healthcare, September 27, 2018.

68. Peter Kolchinsky, "Let's Throw a Patent-Burning Party," *Wall Street Journal*, September 30, 2018.

69. Charles Silver and David A. Hyman, "Here's a Plan to Fight High Drug Prices That Could Unite Libertarians and Socialists," Vox, Jun 21, 2018.

70. Alfred Engelberg, "Memo to the President: The Pharmaceutical Monopoly Adjustment Act of 2017," Health Affairs Blog, September 13, 2016.

71. Phillip L. Zweig and Frederick C. Blum, "Where Does the Law Against Kickbacks Not Apply? Your Hospital," *Wall Street Journal*, May 7, 2018.

72. The Editorial Board, "Sticking it to Pharma—with Competition," *Wall Street Journal*, November 19, 2018.

73. Thomas Burton, "FDA Unveils Effort to Get 'Biosimilar' Drugs on the Market Faster," *Wall Street Journal*, July 18, 2018.

74. CMS Fast Facts, January 2019.

75. Juliette Cubanski and Tricia Neuman, "Searching for Savings in Medicare Drug Price Negotiations," Kaiser Family Foundation, April 26, 2018.

76. C. L. Gray and Robert Campbell, "Lowering Healthcare Costs through Safe Harbor Repeal," January 9, 2018.

77. "New Pathways to Drug Discovery," University of Connecticut, Connecticut Institute for Clinical and Translational Science, September 2013.

78. Brandon Keim, "A New Pathway for Cancer Research," Wired, September 4, 2008.

79. "Disease Pathways: A Key to New Drug Discovery," Novartis, October 27, 2013.

80. John Carroll, "CRISPR Pioneer Feng Zhang Co-founds a 'Limitless' Biotech Upstart with Big Plans for Speeding New Drug Development," Endpoints News, March 16, 2018.

81. Robert Service, "You Could Soon Be Manufacturing Your Own Drugs—Thanks to 3D Printing," *Science*, January 18, 2018.

82. Matt Burgess, "What is GDPR? The Summary Guide to GDPR Compliance in the UK," Wired, January 21, 2019.

83. Taylor Armerding, "The 18 Biggest Data Breaches of the 21st Century," CSO, December 20, 2018.

84. Steven W. Little, "Another Megatrend: Personal Data Sovereignty," The Disruption Lab, The Daily Disruption, April 3, 2018.

85. "The C-Suite Battle Plan for Cyber Security Attacks in Healthcare," *Becker's Healthcare, Becker's Hospital Review*, 2018.

86. "Me, My Data and I: 9 Projects Helping People Reclaim Control over Their Personal Data," Nesta, 2019.

87. Michael Nadeau, "General Data Protection Regulation [GDPR]: What You Need to Know to Stay Compliant," CSO, April 23, 2018.

88. Nicole Nguyen, "Will Blockchain Bring Data Ownership Back to Users?" Enterprise Innovation, June 26, 2018.

89. Carolyn T. Lye, Howard P. Forman, Ruiyi Gao et al., "Assessment of US Hospital Compliance with Regulations for Patients' Requests for Medical Records," JAMA Network Open, October 5, 2018.

Chapter 5 – Doing Major Surgery on Washington: Politicians, Fix the Mess You've Created!

1. Regina Herzlinger and Joel Klein, "The IRS Can Save American Health Care," *Wall Street Journal*, July 1, 2018.

2. Scott Atlas, "The Path to Affordable Health Care," Hoover Institution, Defining Ideas, November 30, 2017.

3. Scott Atlas, "The Health Reform That Hasn't Been Tried," *Wall Street Journal*, October 3, 2017.

4. John H. Cochrane, "The Tax-and-Spend Health-Care Solution," *Wall Street Journal*, July 29, 2018.

5. Hal Scherz, "A Regulation That Protects Big-Hospital Monopolies," *Wall Street Journal*, June 13, 2017.

6. Thomas Stratmann and Matthew C. Baker, "Barriers to Entry in the Healthcare Markets," Mercatus Center, George Mason University, August 29, 2017.

7. Christopher Koopman and Thomas Stratmann, "Certificate-of-Need Laws: Implication for Virginia," Mercatus Center, George Mason University, February 2015.

8. Eric Boehm, "For Hospital Chains, Competition Is a Bitter Pill," *Wall Street Journal*, January 29, 2016.

9. Oliver D. Schein, Joanne Katz, Eric B. Bass, James M. Tielsch, Lisa H. Lubomski, Marc A. Feldman, Brent G. Petty, and Earl P. Steinberg, "The Value of Routine Preoperative Medical Testing before Cataract Surgery," *New England Journal of Medicine*, pp. 342:168–75, January 20, 2000.

10. Peter Pronovost, "Cut This One Regulation—and Save $500 Million in Health-Care Costs," *Wall Street Journal*, April 11, 2017.

11. "GME Funding and Its Role in Addressing the Physician Shortage," Association of American Medical Colleges News, February 6, 2019.

12. Meg Bryant, "Is the Doctor Shortage Problem Overblown?" Healthcare Dive, April 11, 2018.

13. "GME Funding and Its Role in Addressing the Physician Shortage," Association of American Medical Colleges News, February 6, 2019.

14. Ameet Sarpatwari and Michael Sinha, "The Current 21st Century Cures Legislation Is Still a Bad Deal for Patients," *Health Affairs*, Health Affairs Blog, November 30, 2016.

15. Reshma Ramachandran and Zackary Berger, "21st Century Cures Act Will Distort the Meaning of 'FDA approved,'" STAT News, December 1, 2016.

16. Sheila Kaplan, "Winners and Losers of the 21st Century Cures Act," STAT News, December 5, 2016.

17. Phillip L. Zweig and Frederick C. Blum, "Where Does the Law Against Kickbacks Not Apply? Your Hospital," *Wall Street Journal*, May 7, 2018.

18. Matt Burgess, "What Is GDPR? The Summary Guide to GDPR Compliance in the UK," *Wired*, January 21, 2019.

19. Matt Burgess, "That Yahoo Data Breach Actually Hit Three Billion Accounts," *Wired*, October 4, 2017.

20. Taylor Armerding, "The 18 Biggest Data Breaches of the 21st Century," CSO, December 20, 2018.

21. Steven W. Little, "Another Megatrend: Personal Data Sovereignty," The Disruption Lab, The Daily Disruption, April 3, 2018.

22. "The C-Suite Battle Plan for Cyber Security Attacks in Healthcare," *Becker's Healthcare*, *Becker's Hospital Review*, 2018.

23. Michael Nadeau, "General Data Protection Regulation [GDPR]: What You Need to Know to Stay Compliant," CSO, April 23, 2018.

CHAPTER 6 – A DISCHARGE SUMMARY AND GLIMPSE INTO THE FUTURE OF HEALTHCARE

1. Matthew Herper, "At Joe Biden's Urging, Airbnb, WeWork, and Others Commit to Help Cancer Patients," *Forbes*, September 21, 2018.

REFERENCES

Argyris, C., 1990. *Overcoming Organizational Defenses*. Needham Heights, MA: Allyn and Bacon.

Argyris, C., 1991. "Teaching Smart People How to Learn." *Harvard Business Review*, 69 (May–June), 99–109.

Berry, K., 2017. *Lies My Doctor Told Me: Medical Myths That Can Harm Your Health*, Berry Pharmacy LLC.

Block, P., 1993. *Stewardship: Choosing Service Over Self Interest*. Oakland, CA: Berrett-Koehler Publishers.

Bush, J., 2014. *Where Does It Hurt: An Entrepreneur's Guide to Fixing Health Care*. Penguin Group.

Chase, D., 2018. *The Opioid Crisis Wake-Up Call: Health Care is Stealing the American Dream. Here's How We Take It Back*, Health Rosetta Media.

Christensen, C. M., 2009. *The Innovators Prescription*, McGraw-Hill.

Christensen, C. M., 2016. *Competing Against Luck*. HarperCollins.

Cooper, B., 2013. *The Lean Entrepreneur*. Wiley and Sons.

Creagan, E.T. with Wendel, S., 2019. *Farewell: Vital End-of-Life Questions with Candid Answers from a Leading Palliative and Hospice Physician*. Write On Inc.

Deming, W. E., 1986. *Out of the Crisis*. Cambridge, MA: The MIT Press.

Drucker, P., 1963. "Managing for Business Effectiveness." *Harvard Business Review*, 41, No. 3 (May), pp. 53–60.

Drucker, P., 1999. "Managing Oneself." *Harvard Business Review*, 77 (Mar–Apr), pp. 64–74.

Fausz, A., Kirkwood, W., Nickle, B., & Sullivan, M., 2018. *Leading Healthcare Improvement: A Personal and Organizational Journey*. Harpeth Valley Group.

Gawande, A., 2007. *Better: A Surgeon's Notes on Performance*. Metropolitan Books.

Gawande, A., 2009. *The Checklist Manifesto*. New York: Metropolitan Books.

Gawande, A., 2014. *Being Mortal: Medicine and What Matters in the End*. New York: Metropolitan Books.

Kaplan, R. & Norton, D., 2001. *The Strategy-Focused Organization: How Balanced Scorecard Companies Thrive in the New Business Environment*. Boston: Harvard Business School Publishing Company.

Kegan, R. & Lahey, L. L., 2009. *Immunity to Change: How to Overcome It and Unlock the Potential in Yourself and Your Organization*. Boston: Harvard Business School Publishing Company.

Kenney, C., 2017. *Disrupting the Status Quo. Northwell Health's Mission to Reshape the Future of Health Care*. CRC Press.

Kevin, K., 2016. *The Inevitable: Understanding the 12 Technological Forces That Will Shape Our Future*. Viking.

Mesko, B., 2017., *The Guide to the Future of Healthcare*.

Osterwalder, A., 2010. *Business Model Generation*. Wiley and Sons.

Ries, E., 2011. *The Lean Startup*. New York: Crown Business.

Schein, E. H., 2013. *Humble Inquiry: The Gentle Art of Asking Instead of Telling*. San Francisco: Berrett-Koehler Publishers.

Schmidt, E., 2014. *How Google Works*. Grand Central Publishing.

Senge, P., 1990. *The Fifth Discipline: The Art and Practice of the Learning Organization*. New York: Doubleday/Currency.

Senge, P., Kleiner, A., Roberts, C., Ross, R., & Smith, B., 1994. *The Fifth Discipline Fieldbook*. New York: Crown Business.

Topol, E., 2012. *The Creative Destruction of Medicine: How the Digital Revolution Will Create Better Health Care*. Basic Books.

Topol, E., 2015. *The Patient Will See You Now*. Basic Books.

Watcher, R., 2015. *The Digital Doctor: Hope, Hype and Harm at the Dawn of Medicine's Computer Age*. McGraw-Hill.

ACKNOWLEDGMENTS

Although there are far too many people to name and thank for an endeavor such as this, we feel compelled to acknowledge our current and former colleagues as well as our current and former clients. Words cannot fully convey the pride, respect, and admiration we have for each of you.

Walking this path with you reminds us daily that healthcare is a calling rather than an occupation. All of us have been drawn to health professions because we want to help people and enrich their lives. We want to heal individuals while achieving a bigger purpose for our society. We will forever cherish the opportunities we have had to work with such outstanding people. You exemplify the qualities of passion, competence, integrity, and curiosity. And your influence on us profoundly shaped many of the concepts and perspectives that we shared in this book.

To our loving spouses: Hongmei [Aaron] and Beverly [Terry]. You have always encouraged our curiosity, supported our endeavors, and never doubted our ability to succeed. Your unwavering love, understanding, patience, and sense of humor make every day more joyful.

[Aaron] For my wonderful parents, Jerry and Carol. You created an environment that enabled me to feel security and kindness, to know happiness, and to have a sense of belonging. Your boundless love is always with me like a handprint on my heart, and your influence will never diminish. I am proud to be your son.

[Terry] For my children, Heather and Heath, thanks for all you have taught me. It is much more than you could know. And to my three grandchildren, Bronx, Renner, and Norah, who fill any room they enter with joy and smother me with love that is beyond what I could ever hope to deserve. Keep questioning, learning, and discovering. It's an awesome world, full of wonder. Go explore.

We would also like to acknowledge those who read drafts and provided constructive feedback to us regarding this book. Those individuals include Beverly Howell; Frank Huber; Blair Nickle; Bill Kirkwood, PhD; Tim Harlin, PhD; John Langefeld, MD; Richard Taylor; and Kenneth Powers.

And finally, a special thank you to Beverly Howell who reviewed the book three times and took on the onerous and time-consuming task of preparing the endnotes. She did a wonderful job and her support is greatly appreciated.

ABOUT THE AUTHORS

The authors have worked together as thought leaders and consultants since 1994, when Aaron joined Terry on the team of a nationally known healthcare consulting firm focusing on strategic planning, process and system improvement, and customer service. In 2012, they teamed up again in a large consulting firm to assist healthcare organizations with implementing robust management systems designed to improve safety, reduce waste and inefficiency, engage employees in continual innovation, and improve the patient experience.

They have studied and taught improvement and innovation for decades and to augment that, have completed this book specifically focused on disruptive innovation. Under the auspices of Skye Solutions, LLC, a company Terry founded, these two lifelong friends share their research, knowledge, and passion with clients, professional groups, and organizations who are striving to make healthcare healthier across the country.

Aaron Fausz

For over twenty-five years, Aaron has been driven by the belief that health and well-being should be lifelong pursuits for everyone, and that our healthcare system should deliver solutions to improve health—not just treat or manage disease. He holds a PhD in industrial and organizational psychology from the University of Tennessee in Knoxville, with a minor in industrial engineering. In addition to this book, he is coauthor of *Leading Healthcare Improvement: A Personal and Organizational Journey*.

Aaron has helped numerous organizations align and improve their personnel and business systems to accomplish strategic objectives. He has consulted with leading healthcare organizations across the country, including Denver Health, Henry Ford Health System, Kaiser Permanente, Mayo Clinic Health System, University Health Services, University of Texas Medical Branch, Vanderbilt University Medical Center, and many others.

His areas of expertise and professional skills include guiding organizations through strategically driven changes and enhancing business performance, with significant experience in rapid cycle improvement, performance measurement, and behavioral change management. Aaron also has extensive experience in the implementation of technological solutions, as well as in executive coaching.

Never interested in the status quo, Aaron has pursued research and writing about disruptive innovation and how it can transform healthcare for over a decade.

Originally from Kentucky, Aaron has lived in Tennessee, Georgia, Ohio, and currently resides in Missouri with his wife and their daughter. An eternal optimist, Aaron believes there is always a solution to any problem that confronts us.

W. Terry Howell

For over thirty years Terry has been learning and teaching ways to transform our sick care system into a compassionate healthcare system that is humble, respectful to all, patient-focused, constantly learning, affordable, accessible to everyone, and safe.

Terry has a doctorate in counseling psychology from the University of Tennessee and after several years as a practicing psychologist, decided to broaden his skills by doing postdoctoral work in organizational development at Vanderbilt.

His decades of experience include serving on the executive teams of two large hospitals where he helped install state of the art management systems. To make sure these systems worked well he helped coach new approaches to leadership, strategy, improvement, education, employee engagement, and customer service. His goal was always the realization of a culture that was safer, more collaborative, respectful, data-driven, less expensive, and more caring for patients and staff alike. In addition to serving on these leadership teams, he has worked at two nationally known healthcare consulting firms as president of one and senior principal of the other. He recently started Skye Solutions, LLC, focusing primarily on disruptive innovation in healthcare.

His consulting and executive coaching clients over the years have included a wide range of hospitals and hospital systems: Sloan Kettering, Yale–New Haven, Vanderbilt Adult Hospital, George Washington University Health System, Henry Ford Healthcare System, Denver Healthcare, St. Jude Children's Research Center, Hospital Corporation of America, Kaiser Permanente, and Dartmouth-Hitchcock Medical Center, among others. Terry is proud of the fact that he was able to provide content and teaching support at the founding of the Institute of Healthcare Improvement; lead the redesign and development of a nationally respected Lean Academy at Denver Healthcare; teach at the Tulane International Masters of Medical Management program and elsewhere; and serve on advisory boards of forward-thinking organizations.

Terry's tendency to constantly push the envelope of improvement explains his current research and writing about how disruptive innovation can transform healthcare institutions. He is also exploring how he can collaborate with others to find solutions to the devastating opioid crisis in this country.

Originally from Texas, he currently lives in Nashville with his wife, who served as a critical-care nurse for thirty years and has helped him "stay real" as he worked to help others improve the healthcare delivery system. Next to his amazing grandchildren, he believes one of the most beautiful things we can behold is horses running across an open field on a frosty winter morning. Perhaps one never really gets over being from Texas.

DYNAMIC SPEAKERS, TIMELY TOPICS

Terry and Aaron have reputations for being fun and provocative speakers while delivering presentations at national conferences on a variety of topics:

» Harnessing the Power of Disruptive Innovation to Create a System that Cares More and Costs Less

» Disrupt Your Hospital before Someone Else Does It For You

» Tearing off the Band-Aid: Why and How Healthcare Will Be Disrupted and Soon

» The Myth of the Lone Ranger Leader

» The Leadership Imposter Syndrome: Superior Rank Doesn't Mean You Are a Superior Human Being

» Leading Healthcare Improvement: A Personal and Organizational Journey

» Focus, Grasshopper: Curing Your Organizational Attention Deficit Disorder (OADD)

» The Main Thing Is to Keep the Main Thing, the Main Thing

» Building a Learning, Innovation, and Sustainment Culture from the Ground Up

» Why Healthcare Initiatives Fail: Will We Ever Learn to Sustain Improvement?

» The Psychology of Change

» The Power of Scientific Thinking

For rates and availability, visit the website:
www.HealthcareIsKillingUs.com

INDEX

E